How the NHS Coped with Covid-19

Dedication

These stories are dedicated to those who lost their lives due to this pandemic, to the loved ones left behind, and to the key workers from all sectors of life who kept the country going during lockdown. Thank you.

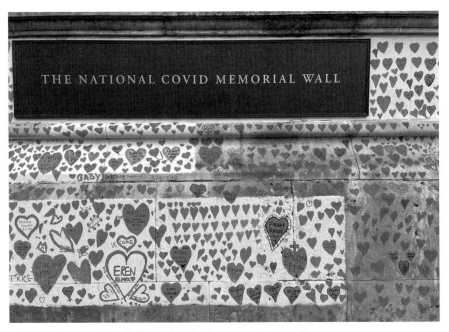

The Covid memorial wall. (*Photo by John Cameron on Unsplash*)

How the NHS Coped with Covid-19

Ellen Welch

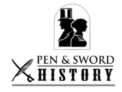

PEN & SWORD HISTORY

First published in Great Britain in 2022 by
Pen & Sword History
An imprint of
Pen & Sword Books Ltd
Yorkshire – Philadelphia

ISBN 978 1 39900 611 8

A CIP catalogue record for this book is
available from the British Library.

Typeset by Mac Style
Printed and bound in the UK by CPI Group (UK) Ltd,
Croydon, CR0 4YY.

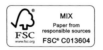

Pen & Sword Books Limited incorporates the imprints of Atlas,
Archaeology, Aviation, Discovery, Family History, Fiction, History,
Maritime, Military, Military Classics, Politics, Select, Transport,
True Crime, Air World, Frontline Publishing, Leo Cooper, Remember
When, Seaforth Publishing, The Praetorian Press, Wharncliffe
Local History, Wharncliffe Transport, Wharncliffe True Crime
and White Owl.

For a complete list of Pen & Sword titles please contact

PEN & SWORD BOOKS LIMITED
47 Church Street, Barnsley, South Yorkshire, S70 2AS, England
E-mail: enquiries@pen-and-sword.co.uk
Website: www.pen-and-sword.co.uk

Or

PEN AND SWORD BOOKS
1950 Lawrence Rd, Havertown, PA 19083, USA
E-mail: Uspen-and-sword@casematepublishers.com
Website: www.penandswordbooks.com

Contents

Acknowledgements

My heartfelt thanks go to all of the contributors to this book, who took the time to pen their stories, during what was possibly the most difficult year of their careers. Thank you for sharing and thank you for being patient with how long the process has taken. I would have liked to include many more stories from patients and staff from all sections of the NHS and social care sectors. Many were approached in the making of this book, but many did not feel ready to tell their stories – either due to the grief and trauma of what they had experienced, or due to the fear of repercussions from their employers for sharing.

A huge thank you to all of the artists whose images adorn the pages of this book. Links to their websites are listed alongside each photo so you can find out more about the work they do.

The mental health impacts of the pandemic are considerable – from the significant loss of life, to the social isolation and economic impacts of lockdown, and the huge health anxieties this has created. Mental health services were already under strain before the pandemic hit, so to help in some small way, the royalties from this book will be donated to the charity Mind.

Contributors:
Jenny Abthorpe, Sam Allen, Neil Barnard, Daniel Berkeley, Alex Bird, Matthew Connop, Lisa Cox, Tracy Briggs, Arina de Bruin, Sharon D'Costa, Alastair Cross, Rebecca Daly, Sonali Dutta-Knight, Brendy Esler, Ines Fernandez Antunes, Michael FitzPatrick, Charlotte Gooding, Jack Gooding, Alex Kumar, Rachel List, Judith McCartney, Gilly McLaren, Nick Murch, Sara Caterine O'Rourke, Randall Ortel, Ellie Philpotts, Jane Russell, Rebecca Scott, Rose Singleton, Anna Startup, Andrew Stein, Elaine Tennant, Natalie Thurtle, Elizabeth Toberty, Emma Tyrrell, Carey Wolfe, Yaning Wu.

Preface

2020 will forever be remembered as the year the coronavirus pandemic changed life as we know it across the world. Economies crashed, livelihoods were eradicated, and thousands of lives were shortened or devastated by the effects of this novel virus. In the UK, the National Health Service was thrust into the limelight as the country watched our healthcare system respond to the consequences of this disease.

This book traces a timeline of the pandemic in the UK, highlighting key events in the way the NHS approached these unparalleled events. Alongside the facts, are stories. Every one of us has a 'Covid story' to tell, and this book is a collection of some of these stories from our frontline staff.

As the country went into rapid lockdown in March 2020, the staff of the NHS donned their PPE and continued to work. They tell us what peak pandemic was like for them.

Introduction

On New Year's Eve 2019, local government authorities in Wuhan, Hubei Province, China, released a health alert, announcing clusters of a mysterious pneumonia in their city. Doctors in Wuhan noticed that many of the patients presenting with this new disease had all visited the city's Huanan seafood market before getting ill.

As the fireworks went off to welcome in 2020, we were oblivious in the UK (and indeed around the world) as to how our lives were about to change. The early reports from Wuhan were barely given a passing glance, but this new coronavirus was already making its way around the globe, silently spreading from person to person, aboard ships and planes. Alarms were sounded in the scientific community as early as January, and a COBRA crisis meeting was called; however, policy makers continued to reassure us (for over a month) that the risk to the UK public was low.

By the time the enormity of this disease was realised, and lockdown initiated on 23 March, the virus had already crept into the country, through our airports, trains, workplaces and homes. Face masks and social distancing became the norm. Thousands were furloughed, while those who were able, worked from home. Schools were closed and Zoom lessons and home schooling took their place. As stores closed in the first lockdown, panic buying set in, with limits placed on toilet paper and hand sanitiser. Sports seasons and cultural events were all cancelled – as were weddings and funerals. Petrol prices plunged (to almost £1 a litre) as the nation stayed home. Airlines were grounded – and air pollution improved in response to the reduced traffic emissions.

The Covid-19 pandemic is the defining global health crisis of our time. It has reached every continent – including Antarctica, and by the end of 2020, the official global death toll from the disease stood at 1,813,188, with estimates from the World Health Organization that this figure could in reality be as high as 3 million, based on excess mortality estimates for 2020. In the UK, 2,656,174 cases had been recorded by 31 December 2020, and 76,401 deaths.

What is Covid-19?

I'm sure we all know more about viruses now than we would ever have wished to know, but let's start with an introduction to the disease that has impacted us all so much.

Coronaviruses are a large family of viruses which includes the common cold, the more deadly Middle East Respiratory Syndrome (MERS) and Severe Acute Respiratory Syndrome (SARS) – which caused a pandemic of its very own in 2003. A novel coronavirus, such as Covid-19, is a new strain of coronavirus that has not been previously identified in humans.

On 11 February 2020, the WHO announced that the disease caused by this novel coronavirus would be called 'coronavirus disease 2019', or 'Covid-19'. The new coronavirus identified as causing the disease was named 'Severe Acute Respiratory Syndrome Coronavirus 2' (SARS-CoV-2).

We know that many disease-causing microbes only infect animals, some only infect humans, and others can infect both. Coronaviruses are common in the world of veterinary medicine – since they affect many domestic animal species (dogs, cats, pigs, poultry). Bats, birds and rodents are recognised as natural reservoirs – meaning, these species carry the virus, but don't become unwell from it, and most animal coronaviruses only infect animals and not humans.

Coronaviruses have a history of transferring between species. In 2002, SARS was transmitted to humans via civet cats, and in 2012, MERS jumped from dromedary camels to humans [GONG, S et al 2018]. The exact source of Covid-19 is still not known for certain, and possibly never will be, but it is known that it made the jump to humans from an animal source (probably bats via pangolins [Xiao K et al 2020]). The first infections were linked to a live animal market where pangolins are consumed as a delicacy or used for medicinal purposes [XING, S et al 2020]. Human to human transmission then occurred extensively, mainly via respiratory droplet and fomite spread. (The virus was declared airborne by WHO in March 2021 – despite their initial stance a year earlier saying it was not – meaning indoor, crowded spaces with inadequate ventilation pose the highest risks of transmission.[WHO 2020f])

Covid-19 is made up of a single strand of RNA (ribonucleic acid), protected by a fatty membrane which is covered in crown-like spikes (which give it its name – corona means crown). The fatty membrane breaks apart in contact with soap – which is why handwashing has been so emphasised. This tiny microbe measures a mere 120 nanometres across – which means a hundred million viral particles can fit onto the head of a pin and only a few hundred viral particles need to be inhaled to cause infection.

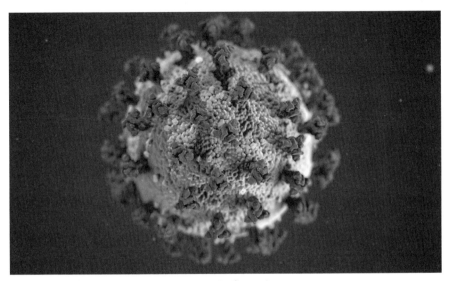

Coronavirus. (*Credit: Photo by CDC on Unsplash*)

Genome sequence data from SARS-CoV-2 has been analysed and compared to known coronavirus strains which has determined that the virus is the product of natural evolution – disproving conspiracy theories that the virus was engineered in a laboratory [ANDERSON KG et al 2020].

SARS (caused by the virus known as SARS-CoV-1) shows many similarities to Covid-19 but did not cause a pandemic on the same scale. It emerged in late 2002 at a seafood market in Guangdong, China, and spread to thirty countries, infecting approximately 8,437 people and killing 813 before it was declared to be contained by the World Health Organization less than a year later. SARS displayed a similar transmissibility to Covid-19 – with each patient infecting on average three other people (the reproduction number or R0), but SARS petered out fairly quickly in comparison to the devastation caused by Covid-19. This can be explained by the case fatality rate, which is how epidemiologists measure the severity of a disease and its ability to cause death. In a nutshell, SARS was more lethal than Covid-19 with a case fatality rate or around 11 per cent, whereas Covid-19's is estimated in the range of 0.5 per cent–1.2 per cent [WHO 2003].

Clinical Features

As early as January 2020, *The Lancet* published the first clinical description of Covid-19. Many patients appeared to have a mild illness and a rapid recovery, but around 20 per cent were not so fortunate and developed severe symptoms. Cough and fever were the commonest presenting symptoms, along with muscle aches and fatigue. Anosmia (loss of sense of smell) was later added to the list of key symptoms. Those developing severe illness typically developed shortness of breath around a week after the initial symptoms and pneumonia which progressed quickly to acute respiratory distress syndrome. In the most severe cases, the infection triggered their immune systems to release a flood of immune cells known as a cytokine storm, which attacked the healthy tissues they should be protecting. Patients developed multiple organ failure, blood clots and secondary infections. The Chinese doctors were clear in January that this new coronavirus had 'pandemic potential' as the number of deaths from it was rising quickly, and stressed that no treatment existed for the pneumonia that developed, other than supportive treatment from a ventilator on an intensive care unit [HUANG, C ET AL 2020].

We've all seen the devastation of severe Covid-19, but at the opposite end of the spectrum are the people who have caught the virus, but display no symptoms at all (asymptomatic cases). Symptoms typically appear 2–14 days after exposure to the virus – 5 days on average, which is why quarantine periods are so important for those who have been in close contact with positive cases. During this timescale, known as the incubation period, people can be infectious before they develop any symptoms, and can remain infectious for up to 10 days – sometimes longer. The more severe the infection, the higher the viral load, and the longer a patient will continue to shed virus and remain infectious [WHO 2020f]. In the UK, people with symptoms were advised to isolate for 7 days which is at odds with guidance from the WHO and other countries. This isolation period was extended to 10 days in July 2020 in attempts to avoid a resurgence of the virus [PHE 2020b].

We now know that patients with Covid-19 can present with a wide range of signs and symptoms. Upper respiratory symptoms such as cough, sore throat, runny nose and difficulty breathing are most common, alongside the classic fever and anosmia, but many patients also experience gastrointestinal symptoms, such as vomiting and diarrhoea, or skin changes, such as hives, chillblains or discolouration of the extremities – known as Covid toe [BMJ BEST PRACTICE 2021].

What has also emerged as the pandemic has dragged on, is that roughly 10 in 100 people infected with Covid-19 will have symptoms lasting longer than three weeks. Many patients have reported sometimes debilitating symptoms lasting for months – a condition termed 'Long Covid'. Common symptoms of this include a persistent low-grade fever, cough and fatigue. A myriad of other long lasting symptoms have been described, including shortness of breath, chest pain, muscle aches, rashes, problems with memory and concentration, and mental health problems [BMJ BEST PRACTICE 2021].

As of June 2021, more than 170 million confirmed cases have been reported worldwide, and more than 3.5 million people have died. Approximately 80 in 100 people with Covid-19 will have a mild or moderate illness, while 20 in 100 people develop more severe symptoms. Predicting who these people will be is not possible, although the infection is likely to be more serious in older people with pre-existing long-term health problems [BMJ BEST PRACTICE 2021].

366 Days of Covid – A Timeline of 2020

Starting with the last day of 2019, which permitted Covid-19 to be given the '19' segment of its name, the key events of 2020, relevant to the experience in the UK, are outlined in a timeline. This approach allows the reader to see clearly how events unfolded, with some commentary and personal accounts enhancing the journey.

31 Dec 2019

A cluster of cases of pneumonia 'of an unknown cause' are reported to the World Health Organisation (WHO) by Chinese authorities [CHP 2020].

The Wuhan Municipal Health Commission in Wuhan City, Hubei Province, China, reported twenty-seven cases of pneumonia (seven severe cases) of unknown aetiology. A common link among these patients is attendance at the city's Huanan Seafood Wholesale Market – a live animal market which is shut down on New Years Day [WCHC 2019]. The outbreak received little attention globally, although later studies suggest that the disease had been spreading through the Hubei province for at least six weeks [BRYNER, J 2020], and may have already surfaced at this point in both France [REUTERS IN PARIS 2020] and Italy [VAGNONI, G 2020].

January

- 44 cases detected by 3 Jan 2020 (WHO 2020a)

7 Jan 2020

A novel coronavirus is identified by Chinese authorities as the causative agent for the cases of pneumonia [WANG, C ET AL 2020].

WHO issue guidance to all countries on how to detect, test and manage potential cases based on experience with SARS, MERS and current knowledge of the virus [WHO 12 Jan 2020].

11 Jan 2020

The first known death from the virus is reported by Chinese state media – a 61-year-old man who was a regular customer at the market in Wuhan where the virus is believed to have originated [QIN, A ET AL 2020]. To date, they say, no medical staff are infected and no clear evidence of human-to-human transmission found. Symptoms of the disease are reported to include fever, dry cough and shortness of breath. Patients with severe disease developed Acute Respiratory Distress Syndrome (ARDS), requiring admission to intensive care with respiratory support [HUANG, C ET AL 2020].

12 Jan 2020

China publicly share the genetic sequence of Covid-19 [Holmes, E. 2020].

13 Jan 2020

The first recorded case of Covid-19 outside of China is reported in Thailand in a traveller who arrived there from Wuhan [WHO 2020a].

16 Jan 2020

As early as January, scientists in the UK begin to raise concerns about the news from Wuhan. Devi Sridhar, professor of global public health at Edinburgh University raised concerns on Twitter.

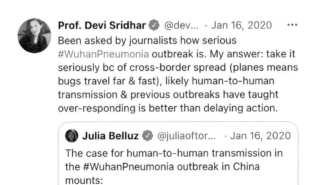

Prof. Devi Sridhar ✔ @dev... · Jan 16, 2020   •••
Been asked by journalists how serious #WuhanPneumonia outbreak is. My answer: take it seriously bc of cross-border spread (planes means bugs travel far & fast), likely human-to-human transmission & previous outbreaks have taught over-responding is better than delaying action.

> 🔵 **Julia Belluz** ✔ @juliaoftor... · Jan 16, 2020
> The case for human-to-human transmission in the #WuhanPneumonia outbreak in China mounts:
>
> A new case turned up in Japan. Like the case in Thailand, the man never visited the market at the center of the outbreak.
>
> vox.com/2020/1/9/21058...

💬 76   ⟲ 1.4K   ♡ 3.2K   ↥

20–22 Jan 2020

Human-human transmission is confirmed [WHO 22 Jan 2020]. The first case in the United States is confirmed [HOLSHUE, M.L ET AL 2020] and Public Health England move the risk level to the British public from 'very low' to 'low' [BFPG 2020].

23 Jan 2020

The cities of Wuhan, Xiantao and Chibi in Hubei province (a total of 56 million people) are quarantined as air and rail departures are suspended. The Chinese Railway administration show that almost 100,000 people had already departed from Wuhan train station before the lockdown [BFPG 2020]. At this point, at least twenty-six deaths have been reported and construction begins in Wuhan for a specialist emergency hospital (which later opens on 3 Feb) [SMITH, N. ET AL 2020].

24 Jan 2020

A COBRA meeting is held by the government on the virus. A team at Imperial College led by Professor Neil Ferguson produced a modelling assessment of the virus, showing its unusually high infectivity rate, which is shared at this meeting [CALVERT J et al 2020]. Most flu outbreaks have an infectivity rate of 1.3, whereas this virus has a rate of up to 3 (meaning each person with the virus would typically infect up to three more people) [IMAI N et al 2020]. The UK Foreign and Commonwealth Office advises against all travel to China's Hubei Province [BFPG 2020].

26 Jan 2020
Chinese New Year Celebrations take place in central London as thousands gather in Chinatown to celebrate the Year of the Rat [SPEARE-COLE, R. 2020]. The WHO reports 2,014 cases globally at this point, twenty-nine of these outside of China, and fifty-six deaths [WHO 2020a].

28 Jan 2020
The WHO Director General travels to Beijing to learn more about China's response to the outbreak [WHO 2020a]. The UK Foreign and Commonwealth Office update their guidance advising against travel to all of Mainland China [BFPG 2020].

30 Jan 2020
WHO declares a Public Health Emergency of International Concern (PHEIC), reporting 7,818 total confirmed cases worldwide – the majority in China, with eighty-two cases reported in eighteen other countries [WHO 2020a]. Declaring a PHEIC means the disease poses a public health risk through international spread and requires a coordinated international response to control it.

31 Jan 2020
The UK's first two patients test positive for Covid-19 – two Chinese nationals from the same family staying at a hotel in York. Britons evacuated from Wuhan arrive in the UK and are quarantined for 14 days at Arrowe Park hospital in Merseyside [BBC 2020a]. British Airways suspends all flights to and from Mainland China [REUTERS 2020].

February

- 11,953 cases globally; 23 countries affected
- 11,821 cases in China; 259 deaths
- 132 cases outside China; 0 deaths
- 2 cases in the UK; 0 deaths
  (WHO 2020a)

Figure 1. Countries, territories or areas with reported confirmed cases of 2019-nCoV, 01 February 2020

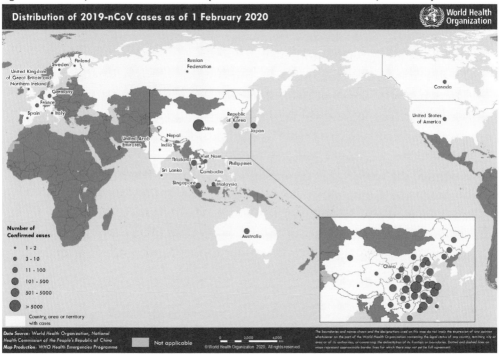

3 Feb 2020

The Diamond Princess cruise ship is quarantined in Yokohama, Japan, after Japanese authorities are notified of a symptomatic passenger who departed the ship in Hong Kong earlier in the cruise. Two days later, all 3,711 people on board are quarantined. Among these, 712 tested positive for Covid-19. Of these, 331 (46.5%) were asymptomatic at the time of testing. Among the 381 patients with symptoms, 37 required intensive care (9.7%) and 9 died (1.3%) [MORIARTY, L.F. ET AL 2020].

7 Feb 2020

Opthalmologist Dr Li Wenliang, one of the first to raise concerns about Covid-19 in China dies of the virus, aged 33 years. He had been reprimanded by authorities in January, accused of making false statements that disturbed the public order. and made to denounce his warnings about the disease. 'One of the world's most important warning systems for a deadly new outbreak is a doctor's or nurse's recognition [of it]', said Tom Inglesby, the Director of the Centre for Health Security at John Hopkins School of Public Health, 'It takes intelligence and courage to step up and say something like that.' His death sparked outrage across China, as people

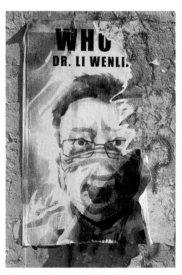

Damaged poster of Dr Li Wenliang (April 2020). (*PetrVod via Wikimedia Commons*)

recognised the truth in Li's comments prior to death: 'If the officials had disclosed information about the epidemic earlier, I think it would have been a lot better.' [GREEN, A (2020)].

Hong Kong introduces prison sentences for anyone breaking quarantine rules [AFP 2020].

11 Feb 2020

WHO announces that SARS-CoV-2 (the new virus identified as causing coronavirus disease) will be called Covid-19. 'Covi' for coronavirus, 'D' for disease and '19' for the year it was first identified, 2019 [WHO 2020b].

14 Feb 2020

Egypt confirms the first recorded case on the African continent. Meanwhile, China reviews its trade and consumption of wildlife, which has been identified as a probable source of the outbreak [BFPG 2020].

19–20 Feb 2020

Iran confirmed its first two deaths from the disease, hours after confirming its first cases. Six days later, the country emerges as a second worldwide focus point for the virus with ninety-five cases and fifteen deaths [IBRAHIM, A 2020, WHO 2020a].

What's in a name?
The WHO created guidelines in 2015 to minimise the negative impacts of disease names on trade, travel and animal welfare, and to avoid causing offence to any groups of people. Prohibited terms included any geographical locations or cultural references such as 'Spanish Flu' or 'Japanese encephalitis'; reference to animals or food ('Swine flu'), and any terms that incited fear (using words such as 'fatal' or 'unknown') [WHO 2015].

When 'AIDS' first emerged in the 1980s, it was known as Gay-Related Immune Deficiency (GRID), creating a huge stigma among the homosexual community. The name itself undermined the public health messages to stop the spread of the disease, since people believed they couldn't catch it unless they were gay. It was renamed AIDS in 1982 [AVERT 2020].

Covid-19 has not remained immune from racist nicknames. Sadly, US President Trump led the way in labelling the disease 'the Chinese Virus' [TRUMP, D. 2020], with other commentators calling it 'Wuhan virus' or 'Kung Flu' [LI, S. 2020].

South Korea reports its first death from coronavirus and immediately shuts down thousands of kindergartens, nursing homes and community centres. The country was praised for its rapid response to contain the outbreak, implementing measures such as thorough contact-tracing; strict quarantine; testing; isolation; social distancing and early school closures. By March, South Korea had the highest diagnostic rate for Covid-19 – a major contributor to controlling the spread of the disease [CHOI, Y.J 2020].

23 Feb 2020
Italy sees a surge in cases (152) to become the third most infected country in the world (after China and South Korea) and ten towns in Lombardy are locked down [THE ECONOMIST 2020].

24 Feb 2020
In the UK, the government decides not to impose restrictions on liberty and movement in the same way as other countries. Instead, they advise

voluntary restrictions such as social distancing, and self-isolation/ quarantine if any symptoms are displayed. Public Health England (PHE) advises against discharges from hospital to care homes. This did not happen [KNAPTON, S et al 2020].

The UK government sends 1,800 pairs of goggles and 43,000 disposable gloves, 194,000 sanitising wipes, 37,500 medical gowns and 2,500 face masks to China to assist with their response to Covid-19. Five days later, NHS chiefs warn that a lack of PPE will leave the health service facing a 'nightmare' [CALVERT, J et al 2020].

25 Feb 2020

Government guidance advises travellers returning to the UK from Hubei, Iran and South Korea to self-isolate on return home, even if they are asymptomatic. Guidance is issued to care homes in the UK containing no restrictions on visits, stating it was 'very unlikely that people receiving care in a care home or the community will become infected' [PHE 2020a].

28 Feb 2020

UK authorities confirm the first case of the illness passed on inside the country. The first Briton to die of Covid-19 is confirmed by Japanese authorities – a passenger from *The Diamond Princess* cruise ship; 800 people are now infected in Italy, and Sub-Saharan Africa records its first infection [BFPG 2020].

29 Feb 2020

The US records its first coronavirus death and announces travel restrictions for Italy, South Korea and Iran [BFPG 2020]. In the UK, twenty-three cases have been confirmed after 10,483 people have been tested [DHSC 2020]. Approximately 442,675 calls are made to NHS 111 in the last week of February [DISCOMBE, M 2020].

Covid on the Cruise Ships

Since the first Briton to die of Covid-19 was a cruise ship passenger, it seems fitting to start this series of personal accounts by sharing the experiences a cruise ship nurse who spent more than half of 2020 working on a ship, without stepping foot on land. Ines Fernandes Antunes has worked as a cruise ship nurse for eight years, and as a chief nurse for the last four. She was onboard when Covid-19 emerged and tells us about her seven month lockdown.

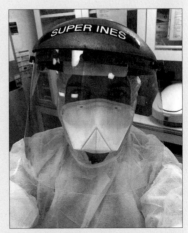

'Ines in her daily PPE'.

"I trained to be a general nurse in Lisbon, Portugal and worked in a variety of roles from the emergency room to nursing homes and also in a laboratory. It was my dream to travel the world, which led me to become a cruise ship nurse. I love my job – every day is different and presents a new challenge.

In February 2020, when news of Covid-19 started to emerge, I was working on a large ship sailing out of the USA, with around 4,500 guests on board. Like many people, I thought this was going to be something that would pass quickly, like flu season. I wish it had been as simple as that! Our first contact with the impact of the disease on board was in mid-February. A family from China presented to the medical facility, asking us to review their child with a fever. We ran all the tests we had on board – trying to determine the cause (at this point we had no access to Covid-19 testing and knew very little about the virus). The on-board tests were all negative, but we treated the case as we would treat any infectious disease, wearing PPE and maintaining strict isolation measures. Several guests on board had travelled from Shanghai or Hong Kong to board the ship and we isolated all of these guests as a precaution. The index case went directly to hospital when the cruise ended and ultimately tested negative for Covid-19.

By early March, I was transferred to another ship based in the Caribbean and the cases slowly started to rise. One crew member presented with an isolated fever, but every day a different symptom

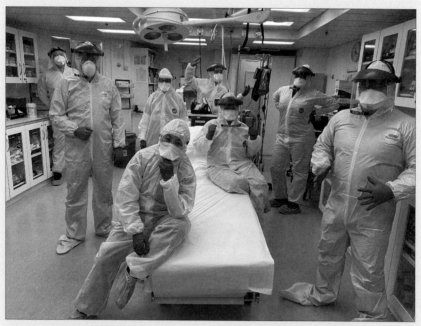

'The Ship's Medical Team'.

would emerge. We considered diagnoses ranging from influenza to appendicitis. After 6 days of treatment, his oxygen levels dropped so low overnight, that we eventually disembarked him from the ship to a shoreside hospital – and he was confirmed to have Covid-19. This was our first confirmed case. On the same day, we disembarked another patient with symptoms of acute appendicitis, who also tested positive for Covid-19 on the routine hospital admission screen. Following this, a huge operation was launched to isolate all close contacts of these patients.

At this point in time, we didn't know what we know now. Every day we were bombarded with guidelines and information about this new disease, and each day we were adjusting our rules and protocols. On 15 March – our six-month quarantine began. Guests stopped sailing and we were isolated on board (at the time of writing I have not stepped foot on land for 200 days). Strict social distancing measures were implemented, with constant face masks in use. The gym, pools and social areas were closed, and meal-times were restricted to no more than two people per table.

Our medical team isolated in our own bubble and stopped gathering with any other crew members. We ate meals delivered by room service in our cabins. We needed to fight against our fear of getting sick and work together as a strong team. As chief nurse I was responsible for ensuring everyone was wearing full PPE every day and staying happy and confident. I also had to ensure our medical supplied were ordered to arrive on time to maintain our stock levels.

The whole operation changed. We divided the ship into different zones, separating the patients with suspected Covid-19 into the 'red zone' and their close contacts into the 'orange zone'. Our team of two doctors and three nurses split up so the 'Red zone' team could stick to their areas, with separate equipment, PPE and constant decontamination.

Since Covid-19 was such a new and uncertain disease, every patient we assessed had their basic vital signs taken, along with an ECG (Electrocardiogram), chest x-ray, full set of bloods and a rapid Covid-19 test (we used the rapid test SARS-CoV-2 IgM/IgG Maccura). Every positive case manifest with different symptoms – some with headaches and fever, others with low abdominal pain mimicking appendicitis. At the peak of the pandemic, we had thirty positive cases in one day (I did thirty ECGs that day!) with over 100 total cases. An additional 126 crew members (the close contacts) were isolated in guest cabins for 15 days and we did two to three rounds of all of these cabins daily, as well as answering calls from terrified crew members. We also had the wider operation to consider: ensuring room service knew which crew members were in isolation so they were fed; briefing housekeeping so that they could clean each area safely; and constantly liaising with the onboard and shoreside management teams regarding our case numbers and management of the situation.

Crew from different cultures had different ideas about how to treat the illness. Those from the Philippines typically believed drinking hot water with lemon would kill the virus. Some crew drank so much of this that there were multiple presentations of gastritis. We treated another crew member from India who started to refuse all medication, believing that only eating dahl would cure him. As this was not available, he stopped eating and showering and felt he was going to die. We arranged for the chefs of board to make him dahl, and we put him in contact with his family, while slowly encouraging him to take his medication. He did improve – but this anxiety and fear was difficult to control. Crew called us crying every day, thinking they would die on board without being able to say goodbye to their family, their anxieties only heightened by being isolated in a small cabin with no outside space.

Many healthy crew members were able to go home (they were not all being paid at this point), but it was extremely difficult to repatriate crew. The world was closed, and no one wanted to accept the transfer of crew from a red ship. The energy of the ship was tense. People upset they were unable to return home when they had expected to; flights constantly cancelled and borders shut. One member of staff had been on board the ship for an entire year. Another took a month and a half to return home to the Philippines due to the travel restrictions.

At peak pandemic, we had a period of a month where we never stopped. Working on a ship is intense under normal circumstances – it is like living in a hospital. Our cabins are mere steps away from our workplace. You are always on standby and ready for action. I would begin duty at 8am, wearing full PPE, then suddenly it was 10pm and I hadn't stopped. At one point I was consulting with a breathless patient on the telephone who called me when I was in the shower. It was common to not finish a meal to deal with a patient. One frequent caller with anxiety called me as I was about to eat pizza – and I recall talking him through breathing exercises, taking the opportunity to grab a bite each time he breathed out!

We disembarked only four patients during the pandemic – everyone else we managed on board, and we had no deaths. Arranging a medivac from the ship was straightforward, but what was challenging, was finding space in the hospitals in Florida for our patients due to the large volumes of local cases. Crew members (as non-residents) were not considered a priority – but they were all eventually accepted.

It was a very difficult time, and some days I felt like I didn't want to be a nurse anymore. It felt like we were in a luxury prison. We were blessed with good food but were unable to choose meals ourselves.

It was delivered to our door on a paper plate, and always eaten cold in between work, work, work. We were unable to step foot on land, unable to hug anyone, even going to the bathroom in full PPE was a nightmare. The housekeeping team were constantly cleaning. Our cabins were fogged three times a day, which made us feel protected from the virus (no one in the medical team developed any symptoms), but it also meant there was no privacy to just have a cry, as we needed to appear strong in front of the rest of the ship.

As I write this, I have been on board for almost seven months without touching land for 208 days. I miss home and I miss my freedom. I feel mentally exhausted but I accept that we are here for the worst and the best in our jobs and I do still love my role at sea. The cruise industry is passing through a crisis and many things will change. Protocols are evolving each day and the way we will deal with patients in the future is uncertain. Routine boarding temperature checks will become common and signing on crew members will be mandated to have certain vaccinations and will have restricted shore leave. Even a simple case of diarrhoea in the future is likely to require 15 days isolation.

It has been an interesting time in our lives for reflection to decide what we want and who we want to be. Helping others and being kind to people is what life is all about: being patient and smiling when a crew member comes to ask the twentieth ridiculous question of the day; or simply smiling and interacting with the servers when going for lunch. I still love my job and I'm proud of everything we passed through. We survived and I realised we are strong. We felt like superheroes at times, being able to help others – sometimes with the smallest of actions."

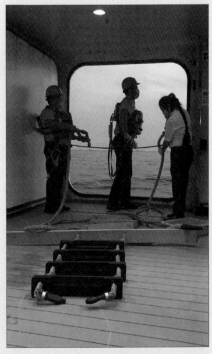

'Preparing for a medical debarkation at sea'.

March

- 87,137 cases globally; 58 countries affected
- 79,968 cases in China; 2,873 deaths
- 7,169 cases outside China; 104 deaths
- 23 cases in the UK; 0 deaths
  (WHO 2020a)

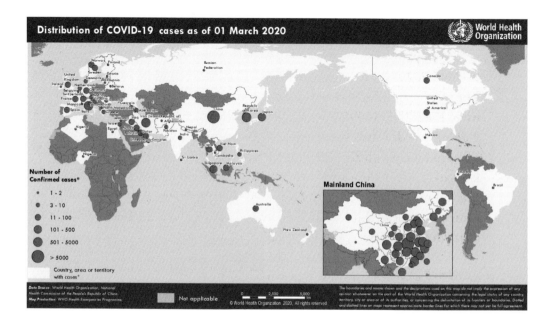

2 March 2020

The government holds a COBRA meeting to discuss its response to Covid-19. Prime Minister Boris Johnson attends, after missing a total of five of these emergency meetings on the virus. COBRA meetings are typically held in response to moments of peril, such as terrorist attacks and other national threats. Despite the official line that the UK was 'well prepared for any new diseases', experts disagreed, telling *The Times* that emergency stockpiles of PPE had dwindled after years of austerity cuts; contingency planning and pandemic training for keyworkers had been put on hold to account for a possible no-deal Brexit. The last rehearsal for a pandemic, the 2016 exercise codenamed Cygnus (which predicted the health service would collapse, highlighting a lack of PPE and ventilators) had been ignored [CALVERT, J et al 2020].

4 March 2020
The biggest surge in cases to date is announced in the UK as thirty-four new cases bring the total to eighty-seven [BFPG 2020]. SAGE advises the government that introducing social distancing measures could potentially decrease the total number of deaths by 20–25 per cent and substantially reduce the peak of the infection [SAGE 2020].

6 March 2020
Prime Minister Boris Johnson announces £46million in funding towards Covid-19 research [GOV.UK 2020a].

9 March 2020
The UK Foreign and Commonwealth Office advises against travel to Italy, while the FTSE 100 drops by more than 8 per cent – its largest fall since 2008. Three days later it drops by over 10 per cent. The 'Spirit of Shankley', a Liverpool supporters group raises concerns about the arrival of up to 3,000 football fans from Madrid ahead of the forthcoming Liverpool vs Athletico Madrid match two days later. A council chaired safety meeting allows the game to go ahead (Spain has 589 cases at this point and declares a 'state of alarm' four days later) [TUCKER, M et al 2020].

11 March 2020
The WHO declares the virus a pandemic, as stock markets plunge and the US bans all travel from Europe (other than the UK) for thirty days. Chancellor Rishi Sunak announces a £30bn package of emergency support to help the UK cope with coronavirus. The Bank of England cuts it baseline interest rate to 0.25 per cent – the lowest level in history (this later drops even lower to 0.1 per cent by the end of the month) [ELLIOTT L et al 2020].

12 March 2020
Advice in the UK from the government is that anyone with a new continuous cough or fever should self-isolate for 7 days. Schools are asked to cancel trips overseas and those over 70 are advised to avoid cruises. Public Health England stops performing contact tracing due to the wide spread of the infection in the community, and the previous advice for returning travellers is scrapped [PHE 2020b].

The Covid Frontline: A Paramedic's Experience

Rebecca Scott is a paramedic in the East Midlands and tells us about her frontline experiences during the pandemic.

"As the country went into lockdown and Covid-19 cases began to climb, we as an ambulance service were weirdly quiet for the first few weeks. Our workload was the lowest I'd seen in the last ten years, although the patients we saw were sicker and had often put off calling for help for a long time. Calls for alcohol or drug issues were few and far between. We were visiting people with a genuine need for emergency treatment who had tried to put off calling us for as long as possible – people with chest pains, broken hips and other serious medical problems who had left things overnight or for a day or two, hoping that they wouldn't need to go to hospital.

The weeks around lockdown were full of uncertainty. There was little official guidance on how to diagnose and treat our suspected Covid-19 patients – what symptoms would they have? Did they all need to go to hospital? Who could stay at home safely? Some of the

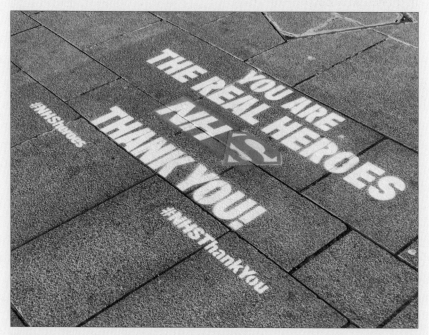

Dr Alexander Kumar – Global Health Photography ©.

stable patients wanted to go to hospital 'just in case', while some of the sickest ones didn't want to go at all.

The PPE requirements changed regularly and eventually we wore a mask, gloves and apron for every job, but this took a while to trickle down through the ambulance service. In the meantime, we were advised to wear different variations of PPE depending on the details provided during the 999 call. We discovered some complications with wearing PPE that probably didn't affect hospital staff as badly – aprons flying up into our faces in the wind, wearing a full-body PPE suit in 30 degree-plus heat, and trying to keep a facemask on while pushing a stretcher with over 100kg of patient and kit for a mile through a park on a hot day.

Our policies and procedures changed every couple of days, and each hospital developed its own system for triaging Covid-19 patients. I went to at least fifteen different hospitals during this pandemic and each one had a different way of triaging their patients and dividing up their departments. While they all used the typical Covid-19 symptoms to decide on their Red patients, some places also took anyone who had been in a hospital or care home to the Red side, and others used additional symptoms such as diarrhoea and vomiting. Even now a Red patient in one hospital could be Green in another. Below is just a quick example of the different procedures we had:

Hospital A: Split between Red and Green ED, but take the Covid-19 patients through the Green area to get to the Red side.

Hospital B: Red and Blue ED, phone ahead with all patients.

Hospital C: Red, Amber and Green EDs depending on the patients age and presentation. No phone calls are necessary except for resus patients.

Hospital D: Normal ED and Hot ED, phone ahead with Covid-19 patients.

Hospital E: Red and Green EDs, different entrances for the first few months but now everybody goes in the same way.

Hospital F: Red and Green ED, phone ahead with Covid-19 patients.

Hospital G: Red and Green EDs, no need to phone ahead except for resus.

We witnessed plenty of sad cases. We saw some pretty sick Covid-19 patients (or at least, patients with Covid-19 symptoms, as we almost never found out if they were actually confirmed positive). One of my first such patients was Debra,* an asthmatic lady in her sixties who had come back from a cruise two weeks previously, and had slowly developed a fever, cough, body pain and shortness of breath since her return. Her breathing was terrible when we arrived, and her oxygen levels were much lower than they should have been. Her partner had also developed the same symptoms but to a lesser degree, and he was able to manage his symptoms at home. We took Debra to hospital – she said goodbye to her partner as we wheeled her onto the ambulance, and I still wonder now if they ever saw each other again.

This would become a regular heart-wrenching scene for all our patients. Before lockdown, most of our really sick patients would still have been able to have their family with them in the ambulance and at hospital, and when the worst happened, their partner or children could be there to hold their hand and say goodbye. But as the virus spread across the country, hospitals banned all visitors to reduce transmissions. Suddenly, families were saying goodbye to their loved ones in the back of the ambulance or as we wheeled them out of the house, not knowing if they would ever meet again. We took Doris,* an elderly lady into hospital with a broken hip as her husband of sixty years cried on the driveway, his dementia rendering him unable to understand why he couldn't stay with his wife. We had to tell a woman that she couldn't accompany her 95-year-old father to hospital after he suffered a massive stroke at home, and then explain to a mother that she wouldn't be able to travel with her 20-year-old son after he had a seizure for the first time.

I went to Eric,* a man in his seventies, for a non-Covid-19 issue. He had been recently diagnosed with motor neurone disease and given less than six months to live as we went into lockdown. He wanted to spend the time he had left with his children and grandchildren, but he was so vulnerable to Covid-19 that he couldn't leave the house and they couldn't visit.

As we came out of lockdown, I went to John,* an elderly man with severe shortness of breath and Covid-19 symptoms. He and his wife Pat* had been shielding and hadn't left the house for almost four months. Pat had dementia and John had taken on all her care by himself, not wanting anybody else to come into their home and pass on the virus. They had only left the house once – Pat's brother had passed away, and they had gone to his funeral a week previously. John had developed symptoms shortly after.

Despite (or perhaps because of) the severity of the virus, we received plenty of calls from the general public for Covid-19 symptoms that were more anxiety related than anything else. It was a mild illness for most people but when the only thing on the news was ever-rising death rates, people were naturally going to get worried. Healthcare staff and key workers were not exempt from this anxiety – during lockdown I went to nurses, carers and even doctors with mild to moderate Covid-19 symptoms, not requiring hospital care but definitely in need of a big dose of reassurance and support. It was a natural reaction to horrible events.

Allison* was one carer I went to who presented with a cough, breathing difficulties, fever and loss of her sense of taste and smell. When we assessed her, the breathing problems were due to an anxiety attack and thankfully resolved just with reassurance – her oxygen levels were perfect throughout. She was so grateful to us for checking her over and told us her story. She worked in a care home with a huge Covid-19 outbreak and had already seen ten residents die from this disease. After developing symptoms herself she had to make the difficult decision of whether to isolate with her two severely asthmatic children or with her elderly parents. She decided to stay with her parents for two weeks while trying to distance herself from them – she was living in one room and using a separate bathroom. Her parents were in their seventies and were dropping off food and drink at the dining room door for her with scarves wrapped around their faces – this was at a time when even the NHS was struggling to get PPE and her parents hadn't been able to get masks anywhere. We reassured her that her breathing was good, gave her worsening advice, and then as our shift was almost over and we still had a few surgical masks left, we broke the rules and left our spare masks with her parents to hopefully keep them safe.

Anxiety hit the patients I wouldn't typically have expected – we went to Kev,* a trucker from Glasgow who had suffered Covid-19 symptoms for a week and was getting concerned that they hadn't yet resolved. Thankfully his symptoms were fairly mild, and his oxygen levels and respiratory rate were completely normal. His wife told us that he was never a man to show emotion, but he cried when we told him the good news. That same day we went to a teenager with a broken leg from a bicycle accident. George* was small but tougher than a lot of grown-ups I've been to, and he tolerated everything we did without complaint – he didn't cry or complain as I put a cannula in the back of his hand and moved his badly broken leg to splint it. But as we wheeled him onto the ambulance, the realisation that he was going to hospital suddenly hit him and he burst into tears (in front of all of his mates) because he didn't want to catch the virus.

There were plenty of frustrating calls too – people who either didn't know or didn't care about the lockdown restrictions and social distancing. At the height of lockdown we responded to an elderly gentleman who was extremely unwell with Covid-19 symptoms. His wife had died of confirmed Covid-19 3 days earlier after collapsing at home and there was simply no chance that he did not have the disease too. We gave him oxygen and tried to wheel him out to the ambulance but were stopped by what seemed like his entire extended family turning up – sons, daughters, siblings and grandchildren. I counted at least fifteen people coming and going from the house, all of them trying to hug or kiss him, or hold his hand as we tried to leave the house. We tried to explain that they needed to distance from him, tried to plea with them not to touch him, but in the end there was nothing we could do and I felt so helpless as they eventually left, taking this disease back into their own homes and families.

Soon after that we went to Derek,* a man with Covid-19 symptoms and a history of severe asthma. His partner had been diagnosed with Covid-19 and had spent a few days in hospital before being discharged to her son's house. Our patient said he had not seen her since she was discharged, but her hospital wristband was on his bedside table, suggesting otherwise. He was acutely unwell and went straight into resus, and probably ended up on a ventilator. He was someone who should have been shielding, and his entire illness might have been avoided if he and his partner had just stayed apart after she had left hospital.

I also responded to a middle-aged woman who had called 999 to be checked over for Covid-19 symptoms – reportedly coughing, feverish and with body pain. When we arrived, there was no answer at the property, and we later found out that she had gone for a walk – her neighbour was a bit on the nosy side and told us she had been going in and out of the house all the time.

In a multi-generational home, I had to explain to one patient in his thirties that his Covid-19 symptoms were mild but he needed to completely isolate himself from his elderly parents who lived in the same house. He just didn't get it, asking: 'you mean I can't even go downstairs to watch tv?'

As we got further into lockdown there were also the patients who didn't have Covid-19 but had conditions exacerbated by the whole lockdown situation. We received calls from people who said they weren't able to see their GP or consultant because of lockdown. During one set of shifts I saw patients waiting for assessments for suspected Alzheimer's, Parkinson's disease and epilepsy – they had all been waiting for months since diagnosis for specialist care. There were the elderly patients who we saw for a range of issues who had rapidly deteriorated, both mentally and physically, due to a lack of exercise and social stimulation while they were shielding. Then there were the frail patients who hadn't left the house for months and had lost the little bits of mobility and stamina they'd had left, and the patients with early dementia who had rapidly deteriorated from a lack of conversation and stimulation.

As lockdown lifted, we started dealing with the after-effects of the virus – patients who survived hospital admissions, only to have to be admitted again with recurrent infections and blood clots. Mental health calls have been rising although the resources for support seem to be more difficult to access than ever.

On a lighter note we saw several allergic reactions with people who had attempted to dye their own hair and tint their own eyebrows without doing a patch test first. There were the inspiring people we met too – people going above and beyond to care for their relatives and neighbours, volunteers helping complete strangers in their communities. We went to Ray,* a man in his late nineties who had fallen at home. He was fantastic – still living alone, pretty much self-caring and very independent. He wasn't badly injured from the fall, and as we checked him over he showed us the shrapnel wounds on his arm from World War Two. Ray told us how he had caught Covid-19 a month ago but managed it at home and had since made a full recovery. In his words, 'the Germans couldn't kill me, so that virus didn't stand a chance'.

It was (and still is) the craziest of times, and this pandemic has brought out the best and the worst of people. There were reports of people spitting at essential workers and breaking into ambulances to steal face masks, but these people were few and far between and the overall support from the general public was like nothing I'd ever seen before. Driving an ambulance means we were one of the more visible parts of the NHS, and people stopped and waved at us in the street, gave us food, Easter eggs and hot drinks, and were so thankful and grateful for everything we were doing."

* names changed

13 March 2020
A multitude of UK sporting events announce their postponement including the Premier League season and the London Marathon, although the Cheltenham Gold Cup goes ahead at Cheltenham racecourse, attracting an attendance of 251,684. Data gathered later through the Covid-19 symptom study found coronavirus hotspots shortly after this event, with cases increasing locally several-fold [TUCKER, M et al 2020].

Portraits and Tales from a Hospital Bed
I began this series of artworks (featured throughout this book) when I was admitted to hospital in December 2020 with post-surgical and chemotherapy complications. One morning, immersed in the daily hive of activity around handover time, I decided to draw, to try and record the united and incredible teamwork I witnessed. I was in awe as I watched how every link in the chain fits together, to bring the care to us, their patients, and during the pandemic, how self-sacrificially the NHS staff worked under great pressure and demand. – Gillian McLaren, Artist. All prints from this series available from: www.gillyartist.com and on Instagram @gillyartist

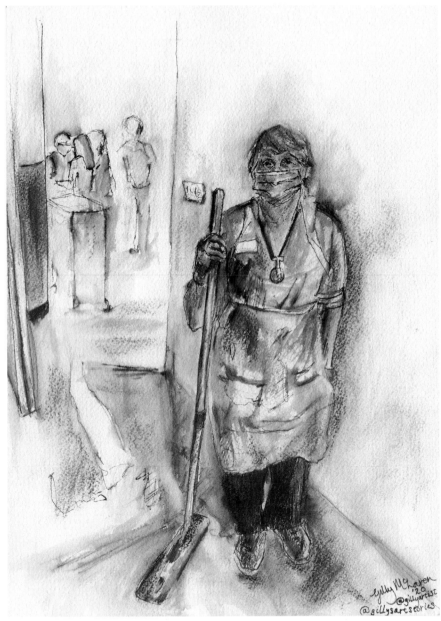

'She brings her own lavender spray – Portraits and Tales from a Hospital Bed'.
This is Margaret, who does a marvellous job cleaning the wards, and even brings her own lavender spray with her, to add a lovely scent to each room. I wanted to portray her, as a vital part of the team (seen in the background) with the light shining through the doorway, spotlighting and celebrating her work. (*Portraits and Tales from a Hospital Bed By Gilly McLaren – prints available from www.gillyartist.com and on Instagram @gillyartist*)

A Patient in my own ICU

Lisa Cox is a Band 7 Sister in Critical Care based at Lewisham Hospital within the Lewisham and Greenwich NHS Trust, where she has worked at for almost twenty-five years. At the height of the pandemic, she was admitted to her own unit with severe symptoms of Covid-19. This is her story.

"I was on nights when Covid-19 hit our hospital, the week of 16 March 2020. We went from a handful of ventilated patients to twenty-six ventilated patients, overflowing from the Intensive Care Unit (ICU) into the High Dependency Unit (HDU) and recovery. We were wearing full PPE and working with partners at Guys and St Thomas and King's Hospitals to make sure that the intensive care beds across south-east London filled up at the same rate, to ensure we didn't have to deny any patients key treatment.

It was incredibly busy. I remember feeling so responsible for all the staff I was asking to double up and work really hard. I recall managers in at 7.30am and still working at 10pm. Staff turned up from other areas to assist our ICU. It was like nothing I'd ever experienced before but like the troopers we are, we pulled together and fought the Covid-19 fight. I ended up working six night shifts in a row to help with staffing and then I had a week of annual leave.

On the Friday of my annual leave, I developed what felt like a cold. I called my manager to ask what I should do. She advised I call the Covid-19 hotline. My partner also had symptoms and we were told to isolate. On the Sunday, I received a call asking me to go to the O2 drive-through testing centre for a test. By this point I felt ill, I had lost all taste and smell, had a cough, upset stomach and I ached from my head to my toes.

I did the test and by Tuesday I was informed I was positive for Covid-19. I was bedridden except when I had to drag myself out to feed my daughter. My other half was just as ill. We were struggling to get fluids down as we had no appetite and eventually, I ended up driving my partner to the emergency department at Lewisham on the advice of 111, as he was becoming wheezy. He was checked over, and staff were positive he had Covid-19, but since his oxygen levels were normal he was sent home to 'ride it out'.

The following day, my friend and colleague called me at home. Tony is a Charge Nurse at the same hospital and we have been friends for over twenty years. He was shocked at how breathless I was. He told me I sounded awful and I should be in hospital! I tried to reassure him I'd be OK, but he threatened to call my boss. I was then texting another friend, Steve, who put it bluntly … If your colleague who you trust is saying go to hospital, what are you doing at home? I climbed the stairs to the bathroom and sat there in tears, realising they were right, but that meant I would have to have a shower. I finally got ready and … drove myself to Lewisham Hospital. I parked in the visitors' car park, knowing the staff one was just too far for me to walk from.

I was assessed at the front desk of ED in my mask, and my oxygen levels were 86 per cent on air. I was moved to a side room and fairly quickly I was given oxygen, having bloods and awaiting the doctors. My own team were aware of my admission, so along came one of my consultants, Richard Breeze. He told me: 'I think we need to pop you on some CPAP (continuous positive air pressure) for a few days, but don't worry you'll be fine.' A little while later while the ED doctor was scanning my chest, Martine Rooney (my matron) and Vik Khaliq, another of our consultants, came and told me my scan showed I had Covid-19 pneumonia. Martine then got Vik to move my car to the staff car park; she couldn't believe I had driven in. They returned and decided to move me up to ICU themselves.

At this point I feel that I should add my other half was in tears. He told me that I had looked so weak when leaving he thought he may never see me alive again. The reassuring team that came to see me left my room raising their eyebrows – they were worried too, and Martine burst into tears. I wouldn't learn this until much later.

So, I arrived in my own ICU as the patient. I did as I was told, except I transferred myself from stretcher to bed. Masks went on, swabs were done, and lines inserted. There was trouble with the ventilator delivering the non-invasive CPAP; they couldn't get tidal volumes, so there were a lot of people in the room troubleshooting. Once sorted it was a blur of vital signs and blood gases, nurses telling me what they were doing and me just letting them get on. I really was a patient; I had no urge to know the numbers or the amounts! Thank goodness, I have since looked many weeks on and I was SICK!!!

I have mixed feelings about being nursed on my own unit, mostly positive. I was surrounded by friends unlike most other patients who were not allowed visitors. I knew I could trust their care, and this reassured me. I never felt scared and I never worried I would die. I had staff bringing me drinks, food they cooked for me, and washing my stuff. I had the banter of friends making me laugh. I also had three consultants a day visit me minimum, and the matron and on one occasion – the chief executive! I must admit I was so grateful I could still use a commode and wipe my own bottom!

On the other hand, I felt a huge amount of guilt. I knew my friends were upset by my admission; it brought Covid-19 way too close to home. I knew how busy the unit was and I felt bad that I was ill. I felt bad for the nurses who had the added pressure of caring for one of their own. All of this has surfaced many weeks later when staff told me of their experiences. One, Sister Toria, a good friend, was told by Vik a few days prior to my admission that the CPAP was working well and that if patients are ill enough for a tube despite CPAP, then they probably wouldn't make it, so when he came to her as shift leader and said he may need to put me on a tube, she burst into tears and begged him not to. Luckily, I responded to the treatment and got better. A few days on I had a shower and that was bliss!

My poor family, I should mention them: the kids were with my ill partner and worried – thank goodness for Face Time! My family in Wiltshire only knew about Covid-19 from what they heard in the press – which was rather negative to be honest. My poor mum who was at home shielding with my dad drove to my sister's house and stood in her driveway sobbing that she may lose her eldest child without seeing her and my sister couldn't even give her a hug! Even my somewhat hard-faced (but beautiful) niece broke down in tears! All things I thankfully found out later. I remember calling people on Face Time and they would start to cry (I must've looked really rough). I remember calling my friends who are also nurses, Donna, Sharon and Bonnie, and they all started crying so I called Joe, my partner, to say that everyone keeps crying; his response? He burst into tears and said he thought he'd never see me again, I'd looked so ill. What an awful time for all, I think I was probably the least worried of all. Typically though, I rushed to get out of the unit, wanting my colleagues to see me discharged. I did so to a huge standing ovation – I wish I'd filmed it!! I wasn't expecting it at all.

I went home to my still-unwell partner and we convalesced together. I was off sick for about three weeks after getting out of hospital, but I was desperate to return and show everyone I was OK. The locum GP put me off asking for more time off work as she had not received any information about my hospital stay and asked why the hospital couldn't give me a sick certificate. She said if I needed any more time off then she would insist occupational health get involved. I didn't have the energy to argue (they don't get involved unless you are off for four weeks) and I didn't have the energy to tell her that I would not be making up an ICU admission with Covid-19! It's been a slow road to recovery I am only just feeling properly like myself and I've been back to work for thirteen weeks now. I've had fantastic follow up, including an x-ray, CT scan and lung function tests, as well as a follow up clinic appointment and physio input! What more could a girl ask for?

On my return to work I ended up doing a local piece about my story that has led to TV interviews and radio interviews and to my being asked to write something for this book. Hoping that I had a positive story to tell and could also thank the wonderful team I work with – they were amazing and I can never thank them enough. They made the worse time in my life a little easier! I'll never get Tony to see that he probably saved my life with just one phone call and a bit of nagging, with a little back up from Steve. I probably would have stayed at home and suffered. Who knows what would have happened? Luckily, I'm here, lesson learnt, my kids still have their mum, my family their daughter/sister/aunt, my colleagues and friends their friend and my partner his better half! Thanks to a wonderful NHS!"

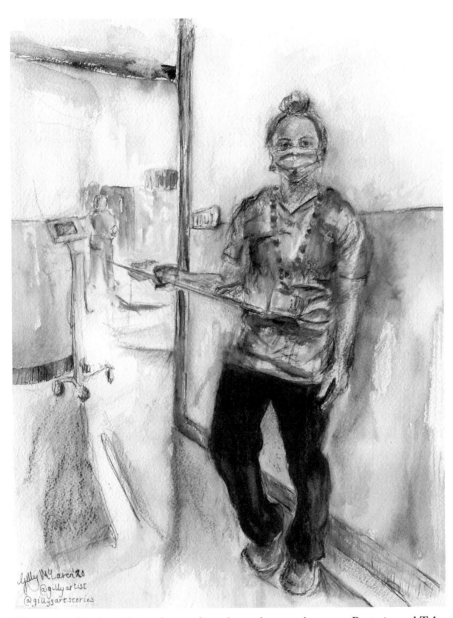

'She wears a love heart lanyard, spreading cheer wherever she goes – Portraits and Tales from a Hospital Bed'.

This portrait portrays a wonderful nurse, Kara, who characteristically wore a bright, colourful love heart lanyard around her neck. In a very stressful, anxious week for me, nurse Kara somehow managed to expertly console, cheer, support and keep bright. (*Portraits and Tales from a Hospital Bed By Gilly McLaren – prints available from www.gillyartist.com and on Instagram @gillyartist*)

14 March 2020

The UK government's 'herd immunity' strategy generates controversy, as the number of UK cases rises to 1,140, with twenty-one deaths [GHOSH, P 2020]. UK retailers request customers avoid panic buying, as supermarkets start to sell out of toilet paper, hand gel and pasta [BBC 2020c].

15 March 2020

Daily televised government press conferences begin in the UK. Panic buying is rife around the world. For the week ending 15 March, a sharp spike in grocery spending and stockpiling is documented. Spending on toilet paper increased compared to 2019 by 134 per cent in the UK and by 217 per cent in the USA. By April these sales spikes had greatly subsided. The panic affected nearly every country on earth, but at different times and to different degrees [KEANE, M., et al 2020].

16 March 2020

Lockdowns begin around the world to slow the spread of the virus. Modellers at Imperial College London find that critical care capacity in the UK will be overwhelmed by the outbreak, and 250,000 people will die unless social distancing protocols are put in place. Boris Johnson encourages Brits to work from home where possible and avoid pubs and restaurants (which remain open) and all non-essential travel. 1,543 cases have been confirmed in the UK, with fifty-five deaths, although actual numbers of those infected is believed to be closer to 10,000 [BFPG 2020]. Businesses are asked to support the supply of ventilators in the UK [DEPARTMENT FOR BUSINESS 2020].

17 March 2020

France imposed a nationwide lockdown as they report 6,500 cases and 140 deaths

In the UK, the biggest package of emergency state support for businesses in announced since the 2008 financial crash, in the form of £330bn of government-backed loans and £20bn in tax cuts and grants for companies facing collapse [BFPG 2020]. NHS England announces that all elective operations with be postponed from April to free up 30,000 beds to fight Covid-19 [HIGNETT, K et al 2020]. A £3.2 million support package is made available by the UK government to support rough sleepers into accommodation during the pandemic [MINISTRY OF HOUSING 2020].

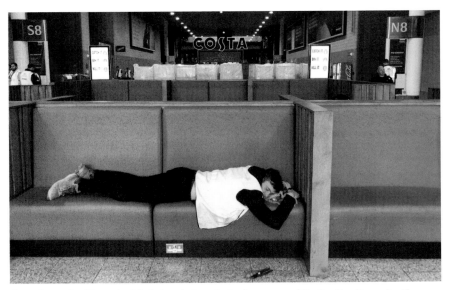

A workman building the Nightingale hospital takes a rest. (*Credit: Dr Alexander Kumar – Global Health Photography ©*)

18 March 2020
The UK government announces that all schools will close from 20 March and all exams are cancelled [BFPG 2020].

19 March 2020
New Zealand closes its borders and imposes two weeks supervised quarantine on any New Zealanders returning from overseas [JONES A 2020]. China reports zero local infections for the first time [BFPG 2020].

20 March 2020
Social venues throughout the UK are ordered to close, while the government promises to pay up to 80 per cent of wages for workers being laid off [BFPG 2020]. Northwick Park Hospital in North London announces a 'critical incident' due to a surge in patients with Covid-19 [DUNHILL, L 2020]. Singapore is the first country to launch a Covid-19 contact tracing app, releasing 'Trace Together', which records encounters with other app users by Bluetooth, facilitating the contact tracing process should a user become ill [KOH, D 2020].

Intensive Care Covid Diaries – 1

Dr Jenny Abthorpe worked in London as a Registrar in Intensive Care Medicine and Anaesthesia as the Pandemic broke. She documented her experiences in a series of diary entries for family and friends, which have been shared throughout the timeline.

In January 2020, I was a dual trainee in Intensive Care Medicine and Anaesthesia with only six months left before I gained my Certificate of Completion of Training (CCT). I had recently returned from a year of maternity leave to my role as an ST7 doctor in Critical Care at King's College Hospital in London. I felt the usual nerves in returning after a year out, but quickly settled back in, enjoying the new challenge of balancing work with a 13-month old. Little did I know about the challenges ahead.

I first heard about Covid-19 at the end of January. Like most people, it seemed a distant threat and one that held little concern for those of us in the UK. As things progressed, I remember feeling shocked at the accounts coming out of China and immense sympathy for both the medical professionals dealing with the outbreak and the residents of Wuhan. I never imagined that only six weeks later I would be witnessing the start of the pandemic in London.

I was attending a course in Portsmouth at the end of February when I heard the news that the first Covid-19 transmission within the UK had been confirmed. The general feeling among the attendees on the course was that a UK outbreak was inevitable but when and how bad, no one knew.

In early March, the pandemic ravaged through Lombardy, Italy. Italian intensivists sounded the alarm loud and clear. Covid-19 was coming to the UK and we needed to heed their warnings and prepare. Behind the scenes at King's, major incident planning began in earnest. The bronze, silver and gold command teams began to meet regularly to discuss and plan the raft of changes that would need to be implemented as the pandemic hit. Our emergency department (ED) had already responded to the imminent threat of Covid-19 and had instigated changes a few weeks before. Frontline staff were trained in donning and doffing personal protective equipment

(PPE) and were fit tested for the special masks required for dealing with respiratory infectious diseases. Our department held teaching sessions on Covid-19, researching and disseminating as much up-to-date information as possible to help us prepare. We wrote, designed and implemented simulation training to prepare for intubating and transferring Covid-19 patients. There was an intense atmosphere of purpose, focus and anticipation mixed with nerves. It was like preparing for battle, but against an unknown enemy. Covid-19 was a novel disease and for the first time for all of us, from the most senior to the most junior, we were all as inexperienced as each other. But this is what we were trained to do, and we were ready.

Our index case was identified and admitted to our first receiving intensive care unit (ICU) on Tuesday 10 March. I was based on the ICU that day and remember thinking 'Here we go'. It was almost a relief that we could finally get on with getting to know this new adversary.

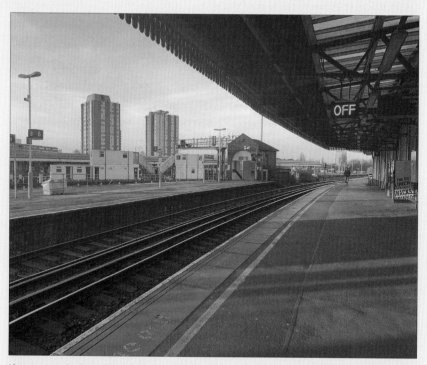

'An empty platform at rush hour – Clapham Junction (one of Britain's busiest stations), 24 March 2020 17:50'.

The following are extracts from a diary I wrote for family, friends and colleagues during the pandemic. I found it a very cathartic process during what was an incredibly busy and stressful time. I wrote much of it sat on a train or platform while on my way to and from work, trying to process and make sense of what was happening.

19 March 2020
I know a lot of doctors are very scared. For themselves and their families. Me too. I was on-call yesterday and spent nearly all of it with Covid-19 positive patients. Some needed intubation and ICU. Some were doing fine and just needed reassurance and good ward care. Some were deteriorating but sadly not appropriate for ICU and were being managed as end of life. They were from all ethnic backgrounds with ages ranging from 20 to 90, from all walks of life and religions. Some ordinarily fit and well, others with significant co-morbidities.

None of them had travel or contact history. I suspect all of them had contracted it from family and friends rather than random strangers. What unified them is that they were all scared and bewildered.

On ICU it's pretty calm and controlled at the moment. Our beds are steadily being filled but we have a comprehensive plan to expand our capacity to 200 per cent plus. I've no doubt we're only at the beginning of the initial wave. The wards, however are carnage. Nurses refusing to enter rooms of Covid-19 positive patients. Physiotherapists not wanting to attend. People using inappropriate PPE as they don't trust surgical masks and Public Health England guidance. Simple infection control measures being forgotten. General fear and confusion, while the patients lie in their beds just needing good nursing and medical care, and their families sit by their bedside feeling helpless.

Any one of us can hold the hand of a scared patient, talk to a family, reassure, manage end of life care and support and educate our colleagues. Let's not turn Covid-19 patients into the lepers of the medieval ages or the HIV patients of the 80s. Please … it's ok to be scared. Follow PPE guidelines, hand hygiene and simple infection control measures. But remember as scared as we are, our patients and colleagues look to us for guidance and reassurance. Let's step up as a profession and be the beacon of light during what may be a very dark time.

Stay safe. Be strong. Be kind.

21 March 2020
NHS England block books almost all of the country's private hospital facilities in preparation to fight Covid-19 [ILLMAN, J 2020].

23 March 2020
The UK goes into lockdown. Boris Johnson announces that people should only leave the house to buy food, to exercise once a day or to go to work if it is impossible to work from home. The Coronavirus Act is passed a few days later (The Health Protection (Coronavirus restrictions) (England) Regulations 2020), giving powers to the police to fine citizens who do not comply with these measures. Australia also goes into lockdown.

24 March 2020
UK Health Secretary Matt Hancock announces that a temporary hospital will be opened at the ExCel London to provide extra critical care capacity – the NHS Nightingale Hospital. He also announces that 5,500 final year medical students will join the workforce early alongside student nurses and midwives [SHRAER, R 2020]. The GMC re-register 11,856 recently retired doctors who also join the efforts against the pandemic [GMC 2020].

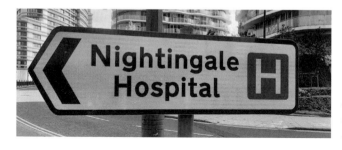

(*Dr Alexander Kumar – Global Health Photography* ©)

25 March 2020
NHS staff begin to die from Covid-19. The first two working NHS doctors die on the same day, GP Dr Habib Zaidi and surgeon Dr Adil El Tayar [BHAGAWATI, D 2021].

Routine dental care is suspended in England, Prince Charles tests positive for Covid-19 and police are given powers to use 'reasonable force' to enforce lockdown regulations. Elsewhere, the Tokyo Olympics are postponed. India locks down its 1.3 billion residents after recording 536 cases. Brazilian President Jair Bolsonaro objects to coronavirus measures being taken in his country, leading to local officials taking action themselves [BFPG 2020].

Returning from retirement

Dr Carey Wolfe was on the path to retirement when the pandemic took hold. He returned to work as part of the Covid-19 Clinical Assessment Service (CCAS). The CCAS was established as a remote (telephone based) assessment service to use the additional workforce mobilised during the outbreak, including retired GPs. NHS 111 passes on calls to this service from patients with symptoms of Covid-19 who require a clinical assessment.

Five years ago, I resigned from my GP partnership to begin my gradual progress towards retirement. I continued to work for a year or so in my practice as a salaried doctor, to help them adjust while finding a replacement for me, and I started doing part-time locums in other local practices. I gradually dropped my other work commitments over the next three years, finishing up at the end of November 2019. I was due to be deregistered by the GMC at the end of February 2020. Finally, I could look forward to realising my plans for an active retirement – completing that long list of 'necessary jobs' around the house and garden, and enjoying more travel, more sport and other hobbies.

The GMC never did get around to deregistering me, as Covid-19 hit the UK's shores. Reports started circulating of retired doctors being called back to help with the expected pandemic. When the call came, I did not receive it, since – I discovered – I was still registered! Despite my revalidation having lapsed, and my last appraisal being long overdue, the GMC confirmed my status, I was immediately put back on the performers list, and my medical defence organisation confirmed I could have extended cover to return.

I quickly completed the online educational modules needed to work for the Covid-19 Clinical Assessment Service (CCAS) (many of which were significantly revised within a few weeks due to the evolving nature of the situation and needed to be repeated!) I used my own home computer, rather than having to wait for an NHS laptop, so set up happened quite quickly for me. The instructions for accessing the clinical software used by the CCAS, however, took several phone calls, several emails, and several days. Judging by the comments of the other CCAS clinicians over the next two months, I believe I was luckier than most to go through the on-boarding process so quickly.

I was familiar with the clinical software used, but it had developed since I last used it as an out-of-hours GP many years before, so I was very apprehensive before my first shift. Fortunately, the e-learning module on the clinical software was updated just before that first shift and made a lot more sense of our task than the earlier effort. The shift leaders were also very helpful when we became unsure.

The CCAS management and administration must have had a nightmare trying to set up a completely new system for a large number of hesitant, 'has-been' GPs, many of whom may not have been used to telephone consulting, and some of whom may not have been that IT literate. But we all know that the key to efficiency is good communication, and a good feeling of teamwork. Someone at CCAS at least clearly realised this, since the administrators who we spoke to while onboarding were very pleasant and tried to be very helpful. They set up a forum for communication between clinicians and management, which proved invaluable – partly because it allowed the early 'returning retirees' (ERPs – emergency registered practitioners as we are called) to inform the later arrivals how to avoid many pitfalls, both in the onboarding process and in the clinical practice of CCAS. We discussed administrative issues and difficult clinical scenarios in post-shift virtual 'coffee rooms', and often came to a very useful consensus.

I hate 'could-have-done-better' lists, but the following are thoughts that come to mind when considering my involvement with CCAS. There was a lack of clinical guidance at the start. This did emerge eventually, but there were several clinical issues where we would have benefited from early guidance, such as rules around isolation when patients didn't fit into the government's criteria.

We were rarely informed of changes in the system before they happened and, more importantly, were never given updates of what was happening regarding the government's pandemic plans or developments. We needed to keep up-to-date with the news ourselves. We gained an idea of where the spikes of infection were occurring in the country from the origins of the calls we were taking, but we often learnt crucial changes from forum posts, and occasionally from patients themselves!

By June, many more doctors had enrolled with CCAS, but the numbers of Covid-19 cases had fallen significantly. It took some time before CCAS started to match the demand with the number of clinicians on duty, resulting in some frustration from 'redundant working' clinicians.

Despite the majority of clinicians being retired, in full receipt of their pension, this was forgotten, and we all had pension payments deducted from our pay, resulting in huge confusion over reimbursement (and no sign of it happening over three months later).

I found my work with CCAS enjoyable, because it could all be done remotely from home, as often as wanted, and it was not taxing, intellectually or otherwise. There were no time pressures put on us as clinicians. The sense of a team finding their way in a new world was palpable and it was providing a service that over 95 per cent of patients I came into contact with seemed to greatly appreciate. As June gave in to July, the numbers of likely Covid-19 patients contacting 111 dropped dramatically, and most of the work was with more complex medical scenarios, which were rarely Covid-19 related. Many ERPs put themselves onto a 'reserve list', in case of significant surges of viral spread, or a 'second wave', or even pulled out of the service altogether to make way for the younger locum and portfolio GPs, whose other work had plummeted.

26 March 2020

The weekly 'Clap for Our Carers' begins as Brits across the UK stand on their doorsteps at 8pm to clap and cheer for the NHS staff working throughout the pandemic. Founded by Annemarie Plas, a Dutch expatriate living in London who had seen similar events in the Netherlands, Italy and Spain, the movement went on every Thursday through the first UK lockdown until 28 May 2020, with appreciation extending to all keyworkers. [WIKIPEDIA 2020c].

Health and Social Care Worker Deaths

Between 9 March and 28 December 2020, 883 deaths from Covid-19 were reported in UK health and social care workers [ONS 2021] – this does not include the many more who died during the second wave. The UK fared particularly poorly when compared to other countries, mainly those in Asia, where with adequate PPE, they were able to get through the pandemic without any healthcare worker infections at all [BERGER, D 2021].

The death toll among Black, Asian and Minority Ethnic people has been disproportionally high, exposing longstanding inequalities affecting BAME communities. March 2020 was a month of chaos for frontline NHS staff, many of whom had to work without PPE. Colleagues like Dr Peter Tun pleaded for PPE supplies only three weeks before he died from Covid-19 last April, while nurses such as Andrew Ekene Nwankwo died of the disease after desperately trying to purchase his own PPE online [BHAGAWATI, D 2021].

Tributes have been set up within the medical community to commemorate the lives lost. The British Medical Association has an online tribute to the doctors who died during the pandemic [BMJ 2021] and The Royal College of Nursing also set up an online tribute to the nursing professionals who have died [KEOGH, K et al 2021]. 'Nursing Notes' set up a memorial to all the members of staff who lost their lives during the Pandemic, and they also pledged to plant a tree for every life lost [NURSING NOTES 2021]. These tributes are welcomed, but it is crucial that a full inquiry into these deaths takes place to learn how to prevent this ever happening again. The impact of this pandemic on NHS staff will have long lasting effects – not only from the trauma of watching colleagues die, but from factors such as Long Covid and the strain of staff being on long-term sick leave.

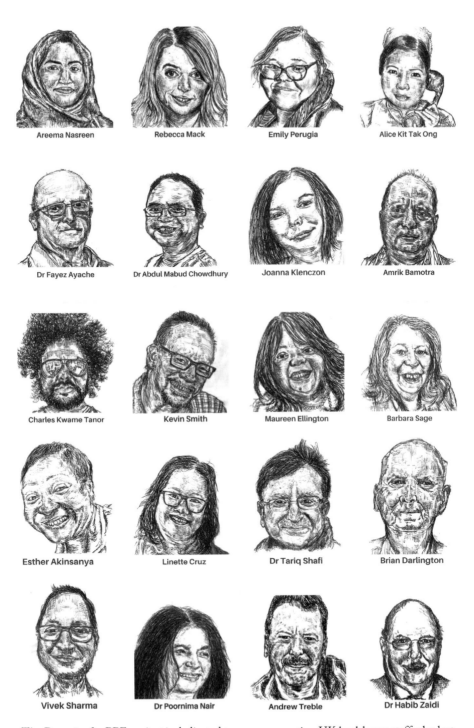

Areema Nasreen

Rebecca Mack

Emily Perugia

Alice Kit Tak Ong

Dr Fayez Ayache

Dr Abdul Mabud Chowdhury

Joanna Klenczon

Amrik Bamotra

Charles Kwame Tanor

Kevin Smith

Maureen Ellington

Barbara Sage

Esther Akinsanya

Linette Cruz

Dr Tariq Shafi

Brian Darlington

Vivek Sharma

Dr Poornima Nair

Andrew Treble

Dr Habib Zaidi

The Portraits for PPE project is dedicated to commemorating UK healthcare staff who lost their lives in the fight against Covid-19. The artist, Yaning, creates ink drawings of each health worker, and shares their stories. Please visit @portraitsforppe on Instagram. The project is linked with MedSupplyDrive UK, a grassroots organisation that supplied PPE to

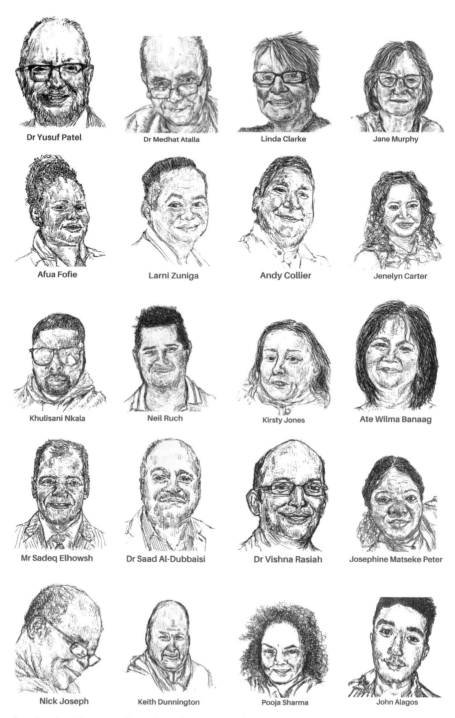

Dr Yusuf Patel

Dr Medhat Atalla

Linda Clarke

Jane Murphy

Afua Fofie

Larni Zuniga

Andy Collier

Jenelyn Carter

Khulisani Nkala

Neil Ruch

Kirsty Jones

Ate Wilma Banaag

Mr Sadeq Elhowsh

Dr Saad Al-Dubbaisi

Dr Vishna Rasiah

Josephine Matseke Peter

Nick Joseph

Keith Dunnington

Pooja Sharma

John Alagos

frontline healthcare workers when they struggled to source their own. They have delivered more than 250,000 pieces of PPE since March 2020 and are now fundraising to protect these frontline workers further through PPE provision, research, and advocacy. Their website is medsupplydrive.org.uk and you can find them on Instagram at @medsupplydriveuk

27 March 2020

Prime Minister Boris Johnson and Health Secretary Matt Hancock test positive for Covid-19. Johnson is later admitted to an intensive care unit in early April. At a press conference three weeks earlier, Johnson told reporters he was still shaking hands, despite advice from the WHO not to. 'I was at a hospital the other night where I think there were actually a few coronavirus patients and I shook hands with everybody' he said [DUNCAN C 2020]. Chris Whitty, the UKs Chief Medical Officer, also self isolates after experiencing symptoms [BFPG 2020]. Over 7,000 former nurses reregister with the Nursing and Midwifery Council to offer their services during the pandemic [NMC 2020].

Intensive Care Covid Diaries 2 – Dr Jenny Abthorpe

27 March 2020

Today I went to work. Ate my breakfast on the empty train. Watched the beautiful frosty scenery go past. Thought about the patients I'd seen who were admitted to intensive care, and hoped they had survived another night. I walked past the warning signs at the hospital entrance – I'm used to them now.

I changed into my scrubs, donned my mask and sat in handover for an update on each patient. Handover now takes over an hour as we have a full ICU. Forty-six patients in critical care. An increase of twenty-eight in a week. Age range 28-70. Most with minor underlying medical problems.

I'm assigned my four patients and don full PPE to enter the 'risk' zone to briefly examine each patient. Switching gloves and washing hands between each case. I touch base with each nurse. Do they need anything? Any concerns? Are they ok? And thank each of them for their incredible work. Every nurse is in full PPE for their entire shift except breaks. They are superhuman.

We're beginning to know this silent enemy. The virus. Patterns are emerging. But it's frustrating and slow. Those patients that are doing less well, we feel at a loss to know how to halt their decline. We focus on the best evidence-based practice and gather advice from regional, national and international critical care networks.

We lost some patients this week and that's been tough. Some patients have been transferred out for ECMO (extracorporeal membrane oxygenation – a form of life support). But we've also had successes. Patients have been liberated from their ventilators successfully, have been discharged from ICU and are doing well. Significant milestones which have boosted morale.

We snatch a few minutes for lunch. So grateful for the delicious food being donated by local restaurants. A definite highlight of the day! The afternoons are hectic. Stabilising sick patients. Proning (positioning patients face down rather than on their back) those who need escalating treatment for refractory hypoxia. Dealing with new admissions. There's now a sense of urgency and feeling of pressure. But we know what we need to do and pull together as a team. Nurses are being redeployed from all over the hospital to assist us. Our anaesthetic colleagues are supporting us too. Critical care is expanding into new areas of the hospital with the contingency plan to achieve 300+ beds.

A new admission arrives at 6pm. He deteriorated on the ward and needs intubation. They're too busy to perform it there so bring him to us. He sits there trembling with fear. Wide-eyed as he stares around him. I don my PPE and go to reassure him. He's exhausted. I drift him off to sleep, reassuring him that I will see him soon. He will be fine and we will take good care of him. He will never be alone, with a nurse always watching over him. He holds my hand and says 'See you in the morning … thank you doctor.' My heart breaks a little. Half an hour later he is stable and settled. I put my hand on his forehead and whisper 'Please do well.' A small plea.

I sit on the train home, it is so quiet and empty. London is still. Londoners have finally listened. And I feel relief.

Its 22:00 and now I'm home. Showered and clean. Sat on the sofa with my husband. After sneaking into the nursery to stroke my little one's head. Another day over. A precious weekend off and then back again.

30 March 2020

UK Foreign Secretary Dominic Raab announces the government will spend £75 million on charter flights to repatriate 300,000 Britons stranded abroad due to Covid-19 [GOV.UK 2020b].

31 March 2020

At the end of March, Spain, Italy and the USA report more cases than China. More than 10,000 people are hospitalised in the UK with Covid-19 and a UK daily death toll of 381 takes the total number of deaths to 1,789 [BFPG 2020].

April

- 823,626 cases globally; 40,598 deaths
- 43,331 cases in the UK; 5,201 deaths
  (WHO 2020a)

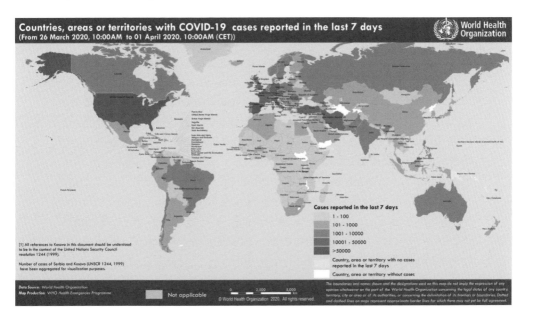

1 April 2020

UK Minister Michael Gove says a shortage of reagents needed to perform Covid-19 testing means it is not possible to screen the entire NHS workforce of 1.2 million people. 2,000 NHS staff have been tested [BBC 2020d]. The Chemical Industries Association go on to contradict this statement, stating that there is not a shortage [PESTON, R 2020].

Diagnostics and Covid
Sharon D'Costa is a Specialist Biomedical Scientist in Histopathology at King's College Hospital.

"I work in the Advanced Diagnostics laboratory where we do further specialist testing on tissue samples. Our work is mostly cancer diagnosis and monitoring, but we still felt a huge impact thanks to Covid. Our workload was affected somewhat due to hospitals only providing urgent care, but the biggest impact was on staffing levels. Many of my colleagues had to shield family members and so worked from home, some chose to be furloughed. Others, including myself, became ill and had to take significant time off to recuperate. The labs were often working with the bare minimum of staff. Most of our junior doctors and many of our consultants were deployed to work in frontline care, meaning that those pathologists who remained had to take on the rest of the work. Even with the reduced workload we were stretched. It's been a real test of our department's fortitude, and we are still dealing with the repercussions of the pandemic: split shifts to reduce staff interaction, hourly disinfection of all surfaces, splash barriers between workstations where two meters distance cannot be maintained, isolation from vulnerable family members due to our work. I think many of these changes will become permanent as we move forward. I'm really proud of the way my colleagues have handled the pressure. It's been a lot to deal with, but despite that we have all (mostly) approached this challenge with smiles and determination, and we kept the lab running."

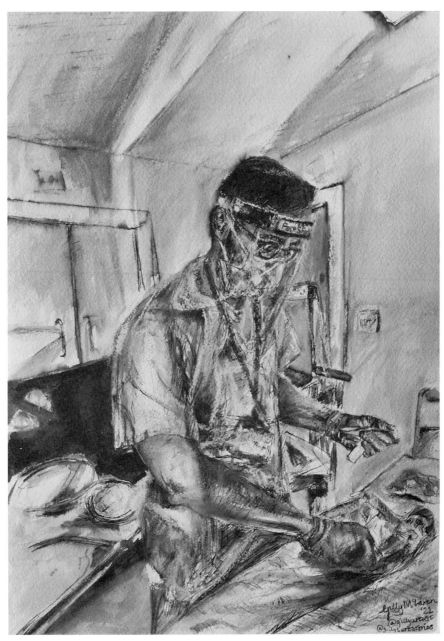

'A Hand to hold – Portraits and Tales from a Hospital Bed'
This is Faid, a wonderful junior doctor who works in the Covid assessment ward. When I was admitted to this ward, I was in a lonely side room. It hit me that a few days before Christmas, Faid sacrificed his own, and his family's health to go to work and do Covid tests like mine. Not only this, he offered his hand to hold, saying 'You can squeeze my hand or shout, whatever helps to get through the Covid test.' And in that moment, I didn't feel alone. (*Portraits and Tales from a Hospital Bed By Gilly McLaren - prints available from www. gillyartist.com and on Instagram @gillyartist*)

2 April 2020

The worldwide total number of cases passes one million [BFPG 2020]. The UK government writes off £13.4 billion of historic debts across the NHS to give trusts financial support during the pandemic and beyond [BUCHAN, L 2020]. Guidance is issued by DHSC for care homes, only now advising family and friends not to visit except in exceptional circumstances such as at the end of life [DHSC 2020b].

3 April 2020

NHS Nightingale Hospital London is opened by the Prince of Wales (via video). Designed to provide care for up to 500 patients requiring intensive care treatment who have already been intubated and ventilated, it is built in 9 days with the help of army engineers, contractors and NHS staff. Further hospitals are planned in Manchester, Birmingham, Bristol and Harrogate to provide hundreds of extra beds should local services need them during the peak of the pandemic [SPENCER, K 2020].

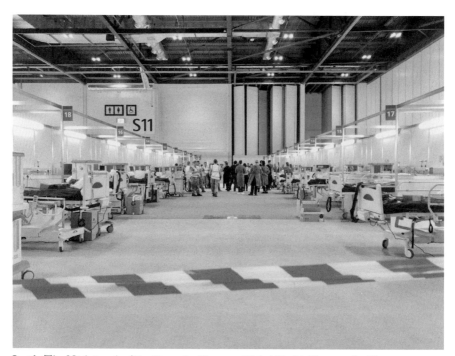

Inside The Nightingale. (*Dr Alexander Kumar – Global Health Photography* ©)

Intensive Care Covid Diaries 3 – Dr Jenny Abthorpe

3 April
Today I went to work. Cycled down the country lanes to the train station. And stopped briefly to appreciate the dawn chorus, such a beautiful sound. Nature giving me an uplifting, almost reassuring accompaniment to the start of my day. 'You can do this,' it sings. The station is deserted. I feel like a lone warrior as I step onto the train.

It has been a difficult week on our ICU. We had six patients die. I can't remember ever losing this many in a week. And I can't stop thinking about the relative of one of the patients who died. An 81-year-old mother, phoning each day to enquire about her son. Her tremulous frail voice and the sound of relief as I update her that he is doing ok. I feel physical pain as I think of the phone call made to her the day before. That her son has died. And the fact that she wasn't able to get to the hospital in time.

As I near the hospital, I join the army of NHS workers starting their day. And feel a sense of pride and belonging. The ICU is incredibly busy now. The number of Covid-19 patients requiring critical care is rising swiftly. Our unit is full again with thirty patients, having received six new admissions overnight. The handover is quick and efficient. The night team of two doctors look exhausted. We give them a round of applause to send them on their way home. Heroes.

Covid-19 patients have now filled a second fifteen-bedded ICU on site. A ten-bedded unit, created in a former high dependency unit area, is also full. There are now thirty-four beds in theatre recovery which are slowly being filled. Paediatric ICU are taking non-Covid adult patients. Two other ICUs are increasing their bed capacity in preparation for the surge. Staff are being redeployed from around the hospital to join the ranks of critical care staff. And we are so grateful to them. The morale of the department is high with support coming from every department and staff level.

The day goes by in a blur. Some patients are early on in their illness and need stabilising, life-saving care. Others are static in their progress and we analyse their numbers and clinical picture, trying to move them forward. Some are getting better and are nearing discharge. We have had some great successes. A colleague and I perform a tracheostomy on a patient who has recovered but is weak and needs slow weaning from the ventilator. But we are delighted that he has got this far.

End of shift. An hour train ride and then cycle home. Two hours later I am home and showered. Just in time to cuddle my little one and read her favourite bedtime story *Spot Says Goodnight*. Precious moments.

It is getting harder to switch off from work. Sleep is slow to come, and nights are restless. Covid-19 fills my thoughts. But a bit of mindless TV and debrief with my husband puts those thoughts to rest for now. Bedtime. Ready for my on-call night shift tomorrow.

4 April 2020
UK road traffic levels are reported to have fallen by 73 per cent since lockdown began, their lowest levels since 1955 [CARRINGTON, D 2020].

5 April 2020
Scotland's Chief Medical Officer, Catherine Calderwood, resigns from her position after going against her own 'Stay at home' advice and is pictured visiting her second home. Boris Johnson is admitted to hospital. [BFPG 2020].

6 April 2020
Boris Johnson is taken into intensive care. The UK Covid-19 death toll exceeds 5,000, with almost 52,000 reported cases [BFPG 2020, WHO 2020a].

10 April 2020
China intensifies screening of asymptomatic Covid-19 cases in an attempt to prevent a second wave of infection, while the number of confirmed deaths worldwide passes 100,000. [BFPG 2020].

The Students Stepped Up
Dr Andrew Stein is a consultant nephrologist and general physician in Coventry.

"At the start of the Covid-19 surge, one bright April day, I found myself walking from the car park (all free!) to the hospital surrounded by over thirty final year medical students. Students using a staff car park! What next? How could that be? They chatted quietly. It was nice to see a smile too. I suddenly realised who they were and why they were there. They were about to start their first day acting up as junior doctors, like the cavalry coming over the hill. Medical students from lower year groups also joined in the effort and were about to start work as support workers and porters.

The wards were grim at this point with nearly all the patients having Covid-19. Intensive care was full – all Covid-19. 30 patients were being ventilated on a cardiology ward. It was getting worse day by day. Morale was flagging but no one suggested throwing the towel in. We were so pleased to see the students. Reports were coming through about outbreaks ripping through haemodialysis units with high mortality. Everyone was frightened, including me.

I had a speech prepared for them, which included the line: 'This is your Belsen.' London medical students worked at the Nazi concentration camp soon after the gates were opened. My mother, a post-war doctor, knew some of them. My speech wasn't necessary. They just went quietly to the wards they were allocated, and started work, including weekends (though remember the weekend and holidays soon stopped existing).

On ward rounds, they kept me back from the Covid-19 patients, aware of my advancing age. One day, a student blocked my path into the side room of an elderly lady with dementia dying of Covid-19. Normally I would have held her hand and asked her if she was in pain or distressed. 'She is dying,' I was told, 'you cannot help, we will deal with it.' I felt they liked to see the patients but were happy if we were 'just there' (i.e. in our offices, waiting to be consulted if necessary). The younger consultants continued to work alongside them in the emergency department.

The students were incredibly helpful, both as doctors and support workers, and raised our morale. The country should be grateful to, and proud of, these young men and women. They showed huge bravery and met the challenge as much as those medical students did in Belsen, long ago."

Intensive Care Covid Diaries 4 – Dr Jenny Abthorpe

April 14

This week I went to work and completed a set of night shifts like no other I have experienced before.

I arrived for my shifts with a sense of foreboding, very aware that the peak of the pandemic draws ever closer. At the start of each shift, I join the critical outreach team for their handover. It is staggering. Approximately twenty to forty patients on the list each night. All Covid-19 positive or suspected. And all on 60 per cent oxygen or more. Those on less get discharged from the list! The new 'normal'.

We are proning awake patients on the ward. Some patients are getting CPAP (continuous positive airway pressure-a form of breathing support for those who can breathe themselves but need help). Some are on 15 litres of oxygen, unable to be weaned down. All are being reviewed regularly during the day by the outreach team led by an ICU consultant. Many patients are sick but stable, some are improving and a few give us cause for concern. The night team will work tirelessly all night to make sure that every patient is seen and safe. Over the week, one or two deteriorating patients are intubated each night and taken to one of the ICUs.

The bleep I hold is the outward facing bleep and covers referrals from ED – all critically ill medical and surgical patients, all trauma calls and cardiac arrests. I also provide support and advice to any of the residents and Specialist Registrars on the units. And the number of units has expanded over the past weeks with ventilated patients in newly designated critical care areas. As of last week, there is also a resident ICU consultant on call, absolute godsend!

Multiple ED referrals are received throughout each night. Majority are suspected Covid-19 patients and profoundly hypoxic (low in oxygen). The biggest challenge is trying to provide patient-centred care when each patient presenting is identical to each other – hypertensive +\- diabetic +\- raised BMI with cough, fever, hypoxia and respiratory distress. They blur into one. But what strikes me is that most are surprisingly calm. There is little surprise when I tell them that we think they have coronavirus and may need to go on a ventilator. Just quiet acceptance. I make many phone-calls to families from ED, hating the thought of them seeing their relative taken away and not hearing any news. I update them on their relative's progress and gain vital information on their loved one's baseline. Information that has important bearing on their treatment escalation. The emotion down the phone is tangible. But the families are so grateful for any news and grateful that we will take them to ICU if needed. Not all need it now, but most do.

I call the family of an 80-year-old man. His wife tells me she is a retired nurse of thirty-five years. In between sobs, she expresses her gratitude for the care we are giving. I feel so choked up, I can barely say anything. It's humbling. I promise her I will deliver a message to him. And I do. We hold hands for a moment as I whisper the words she told me to tell him. He nods and smiles. He tells me he does not want to come to ICU. Two days later, he passes away on the ward, having seen his family for the final time.

But the referrals are not just Covid-19 related. We have a code red HEMS (helicopter emergency medical service) trauma come in. A young man who has jumped from a significant height, his injuries are devastating. Two patients are referred with low GCS (unconscious) who we discover have had catastrophic brain haemorrhages. One dies in ED with their family around them, the other goes to the ICU for prognostication and possible organ donation. Four out-of-hospital cardiac arrests come in, three of whom survive with potential for full recovery. One recreational drug overdose. A urosepsis with septic shock and multi-organ failure. The ED team and phenomenal Advanced Critical Care Practitioners (ACCPs) provide fantastic support. Working with me to stabilise each patient, keeping me fed and watered throughout the nights with their usual high-end banter, ensuring all of our morale is kept high. It is not very busy in Resus but those that come in are super sick. It is time-consuming and intense.

But I feel relief, all of these cases are ICU bread and butter. But the difference is, they may all have Covid-19, so it's all done wearing PPE. For hours on end. There are huge communication challenges. It's distracting. The glare from the visors makes putting in endotracheal tubes and lines challenging. And having to wear sterile gowns, gloves etc over the PPE makes it hot and sweaty work. There are times I want to scream and just rip the mask off. My nose is bruised, my cheeks sore. Even when I am finally at home, lying in bed, trying to sleep … I still feel the sensation of a mask on my face.

Meanwhile, in the ICUs, the doctors and nurses on each unit work tirelessly all night. So many sick patients. The consultant and I attend many emergencies on the Covid units throughout the nights. A number of cardiac arrests. Some ventilator emergencies. We lose patients. The phone-calls to the relatives are like a kick in the stomach. The grief down the phone is heartbreaking and I struggle to hold it in myself, voice breaking as I tell another family 'I'm so sorry.' It feels so inadequate.

But there are many getting better including my patient from the other week. He's doing really well and I'm so relieved. Each patient that beats this terrible disease needs to be remembered and celebrated. As do those who sadly lose their battle.

The nurses in particular are struggling. They feel like they are fighting fires all the time and not able to give the standard of care they usually do. But what they are achieving is superhuman. And still they keep going. We all do. The incredible anaesthetists now part of the ICU family, the unflappable and highly skilled ACCPs, the fantastic ED doctors, the superb and awe-inspiring medical doctors on the wards, the wonderful ward nurses, the doctors and nurses from other specialties now deployed to critical care, the Health Care Assistants and cleaners, the GPs, physiotherapists, pharmacists, mortuary workers, the bereavement office … we all keep going. Because we are the NHS. Because our patients and country need us. And in the future we will say 'we were there', but who knows what the toll on us will be.....

And now I'm home. Enjoying a long Easter bank holiday. Feeling both blessed and guilty for being off. Resting and recuperating for the week ahead.

11 April 2020

Personal Protective Equipment (PPE) and the lack of it has remained a concern for frontline workers throughout the pandemic, with many improvising their own due to short supplies. UK Home Secretary Priti Patel says 'sorry if people feel there have been failings' in the provision of kit [PARVEEN, N 2020].

12 April 2020

The number of people in the UK who died in hospital of Covid-19 passes 10,000. Boris Johnson is discharged from hospital [BBC 2020e].

14 April 2020

Mobile phone operators report more than twenty arson attacks on mobile phone masts in the UK. The surge in attacks are thought to be caused by conspiracy theories which falsely claim that 5G networks have caused Covid-19 [KELION, L 2020].

15 April 2020

Confirmed Covid-19 infections pass 2 million worldwide [WHO 2020a]. Donald Trump, whose own handling of the pandemic was questionable, cuts WHO funding claiming the organisation 'failed in its basic duty' in its response to Covid-19. The US is the largest single funder of WHO. Bill Gates, the second largest, criticised Trump's decision by tweeting: 'Halting funding for the WHO during a world health crisis is as dangerous as it sounds. Their work is slowing the spread of Covid-19 and if that work is stopped no other organisation can replace them' [BBC 2020f].

In the UK, concerns are raised that the official death toll for Covid-19 only accounts for those who died in hospital [MCINTYRE, N 2020]. Testing begins in care homes. The Office for National Statistics indicates that more than 16,000 deaths were recorded in the week ending 3 April – 6,000 higher than the average for that time of year [TRIGGLE, N 2020].

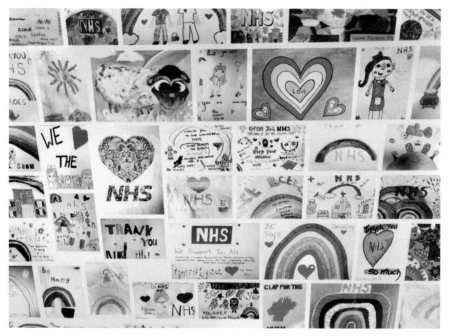

Thank You NHS drawings on display at The London Nightingale Hospital Image credit: Dr Alexander Kumar – Global Health Photography (c)

16 April 2020

Tom Moore, a 99-year-old war veteran raises over £25million for NHS Charities Together by completing 100 laps of his garden. He goes on to raise a total of £33 million which is used by the 241 member charities to support NHS patients, staff and volunteers funding schemes such as bereavement support and staff counselling, and technology to connect those isolated in hospital with their loved ones [NHS CHARITIES TOGETHER 2021].

17 April 2020

The WHO emphasises that there is no evidence to prove whether someone who has recovered from Covid-19 is immune from the disease [WHO 2020a]. Death registrations in the UK are at 207 per cent of the five-year average this week, with 21,805 deaths registered – Covid-19 is mentioned in 8,730 of these [ONS 2020b].

18 April 2020

The UK government briefing reports that the virus appears to have a 'disproportionate impact' on Black Asian and minority ethnic communities and Public Health England is asked to investigate [NHS CONFEDERATION 2020]. Care England, the UKs largest care home representative body estimates that up to 7,500 care home residents may have died due to Covid-19 compared to the official figure of 1400 [BLACKALL, M 2020].

Intensive Care Covid Diaries 5 – Dr Jenny Abthorpe

19 April
This week I completed a second set of night shifts. My second in two weeks. My first two were locum shifts covering for colleagues off sick, providing senior cover on some of the main ICUs. My second two were covering the outward facing bleep taking emergency referrals from ED.

My goodness what a difference a week makes.

This week, there was a noticeable drop in numbers of Covid-19 patients presenting to our hospital and a significant downtrend in those needing ICU, although there still are patients being admitted. ED was scarily quiet.

I reflect on my night shift on Tuesday 7 April, one of the worst I have ever done, marked forever in my mind. There was a point that night that I had a moment of panic, thinking that if things got much worse, we would not be able to cope. In hindsight, what we were experiencing that week was the peak of the pandemic. And we coped and got through it.

Between 27 Feb to 15 April, a six-week timeframe, my hospital had dealt with around 2,000 Covid-19 admissions; 243 admitted to critical care beds (not all of these to the ICUs); 1,210 patients have been discharged alive, sixty-four from critical care. Phenomenal numbers.

My first night was on my usual base unit. It has been receiving Covid-19 patients since day one of the pandemic. Staffed by battle-fatigued nurses and doctors, still deep in the fight against the disease. Morale remains high but it is clear that the past five weeks have taken their toll on everyone. Particularly as we are now caring for more healthcare workers, struck down in the line of duty. It is incredibly sobering.

After handover, we allocate patients and get to work. Reviewing and assessing each patient to ensure they have a smooth night and that they are reaching the daily targets set by the day team.

But nothing goes as planned. Covid-19 is an unpredictable disease but does seem to have a temporal element. Late afternoon and the night are common times for patients to deteriorate, usually coinciding with high spikes in fever. In a few cases, even as high as 42C.

With the spike in temperature, oxygen demand dramatically rises, but is unable to be matched by its delivery through damaged and inflamed lungs, and manifests as a significant drop in oxygen levels. A number of patients require proning to improve oxygen delivery, a procedure that is high risk and labour intensive particularly at night. In other patients, proning does not work and all we can do is support their organs, aggressively cool them and hope they can ride it out. If they become refractory to all oxygenation therapies, the final therapy is ECMO. Sadly many patients are not candidates for ECMO for a variety of appropriate reasons. There are many other reasons why patients may deteriorate, so we need to work quickly through a list of differential diagnoses. Thinking about the usual ICU culprits, but also the nuances of Covid-19 infection. While it is a devastating illness, it is also fascinating and unlike anything I have dealt with before.

Approximately a third of patients on the unit are doing well, gradually improving with a glimmer of hope that they will beat this terrible disease and leave the ICU. Another third seem stuck. Still on mechanical ventilatory support. Still requiring kidney support and sometimes blood pressure support. And on a decent percentage of inspired oxygen. We can only hope that all these patients need is time. The final third are not doing well. On high amounts of organ support. Some on the maximum amount of oxygen we can deliver, but still they hold on. Everyone willing them to keep fighting and praying they turn the corner. It is a worrying time for us but utterly heartbreaking for the families. The only contact they get is daily updates via phone and online e-visiting via iPads.

At around 11pm, I phone a patient's wife. He is relatively young, usually well, and has two young children. His wife is understandably incredibly anxious and has already phoned the unit a number of times tonight. My heart reaches out to her. I phone her, hoping to provide some comfort and reassurance. We chat for around twenty minutes. She is on her own having sent her children away to a relative. She can't eat or sleep. She is living a recurring nightmare. There is very little I can say to reassure her other than we won't give up on him. That we will continue to give our all to get him through this. He is one of the sickest patients on our unit. His body almost overwhelmed by the virus. But he is holding on. I can't give her false hope, but I can give her some hope. I tell her to try and rest. That I will call her if I am concerned. It is all I can do.

The rest of the night is spent troubleshooting ventilatory issues, tweaking medication, adjusting targets and ensuring each patient is stable for handover the next morning. I even manage a bit of teaching on ventilators for my junior colleagues, all bar two have been redeployed from other specialities and this is their first experience of ICU. Baptism of fire!

One patient who had a wobble at the start of the night seems to be significantly improving. Has he turned the corner? It looks like it and I feel emboldened. Hopefully one more to beat Covid-19.

And then it's morning. We do a walk round handover with the day team. The 'Covid Tactical Commander' pops in for an update of events overnight. He looks pleasantly surprised at my reply to his question regarding how our night had been … 'it was a good night' is my reply. He smiles wearily and says that it is refreshing to hear it. And it honestly was. All patients survived the night. Morale was good and our team provided excellent care under difficult circumstances. I feel proud of my department. And I feel hopeful for the NHS. Lockdown is working. The British public are behind us. Every time a new challenge arises, people step up.

But I am so aware that this is not the end. We have a long way to go and many challenges ahead. And while Covid-19 admissions decrease rapidly via ED and the wards, the ICUs will be busy with Covid-19 for a long time yet. Many patients continue to fight for their lives. There will be more losses. We must not forget those still fighting, their families or the staff caring for them.

20 April 2020

Early data suggests only 2–3 per cent of the population has been infected with Covid-19 according to WHO, meaning a large proportion of people remain susceptible [BOSELEY, S 2020]. The number of people hospitalised with Covid-19 has begun to fall in Scotland, Wales and

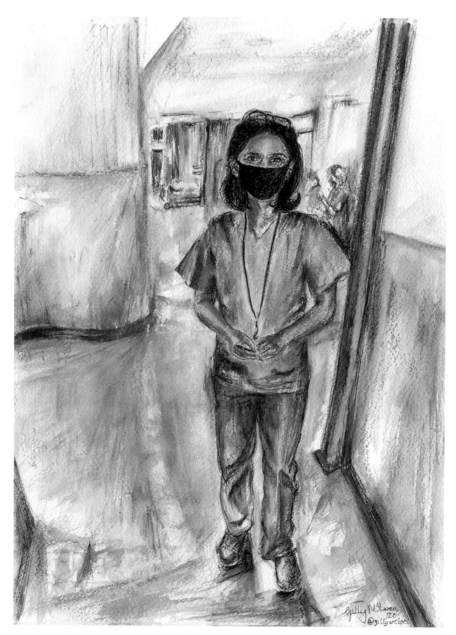

She's simply a hero – Portraits and Tales from a Hospital Bed.

This is my incredible consultant Dorin. It's hard to know how to put into words all she's done for me. She works so hard behind the scenes to bring the best possible care, always going the extra mile and giving me so much of her time, countless pearls of wisdom, kind advice and warm, personal touches to cheer me along this unknown journey. She's always there for me and she's a shining example of such a self-sacrificial person, giving everything she can for her patients. (*By Gilly McLaren – prints available from www.gillyartist.com and on Instagram @gillyartist*)

every region of England [Centre for Evidence-Based Medicine 2020].
Italy and Spain also report falls in their daily death tolls [BFPG 2020].

21 April 2020

The World Food Programme warns that the number of people suffering
from acute hunger could surpass 250 million by the end of the year due
to the pandemic [WFP 2020]. Deaths in England and Wales reach a
twenty-year high according to figures released by the Office for National
Statistics [ONS 2020b].

22 April 2020

Matt Hancock states in Commons that 'we are at the peak' of the
pandemic, but social distancing measures cannot be relaxed. Professor
Chris Whitty says the UK will have to live with some form of social
distancing for at least the rest of the year [NHS PROVIDERS 2020].

23 April 2020

The first human trials of a Covid-19 vaccine in Europe begin in Oxford
[OXFORD VACCINE GROUP 2020]. Matt Hancock announces that
all key workers and their household are eligible for Covid-19 tests, which
can be booked through the government website and conducted at drive
through centres (ninety-two across the country) or via home testing kits.
Hancock also announces plans to restart contact tracing, by recruiting
18,000 staff to assist Public Health England [NHS PROVIDERS
2020].

25 April 2020

The number of recorded deaths in the UK reaches 20,319. Worldwide,
this figure is 200,000 [WHO 2020a]. Figures show that ED attendances
are half their usual level, raising concerns that people are putting off
going to hospital due to Covid-19 fears [MCCONKEY, R et al 2020].

27 April 2020

The UK government announces that the families of healthcare workers
who die due to Covid-19 contracted during frontline work, will be
entitled to a payment of £60,000. The benefits of social distancing take
effect with 360 deaths recorded – the lowest rise in four weeks [NHS
PROVIDERS 2020].

29 April 2020

Official figures in the UK start to include deaths in care homes and the community, meaning the number of recorded deaths increases by 3,811, to account for deaths occurring outside of hospital since 2 March [NHS PROVIDERS 2020].

30 April 2020

Boris Johnson announces that the UK is 'past the peak' and that he will set out plans for easing lockdown next week [NHS PROVIDERS 2020].

May

- 3,175,207 cases globally; 224,172 deaths
- 181,411 cases in the UK; 29,109 deaths
  (WHO 2020a, GOV.UK 2021)

Figure 1. Number of confirmed COVID-19 cases reported in the last seven days by country, territory or area, 25 April to 1 May*

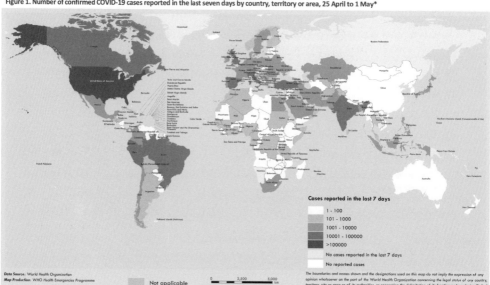

1 May 2020

Donald Trump claims there is evidence that Covid-19 originated in a Chinese lab [BBC 2020b]. Scientists have disproved this theory many times over [CALISHER C et al 2020] and the US have not provided the evidence they claim to have. To date there are eleven independently published studies from around the world that have determined the virus came from animals. Notably, there are no published studies that have been able to contradict these findings or suggest otherwise [MCLAUGHLIN A 2020].

2 May 2020

£72 million of funding is to be made available to vulnerable people in the UK including victims of domestic violence and modern slavery who have suffered during the lockdown restrictions [BBC 2020g].

3 May 2020

An NHS Contact tracing app, aiming to limit a second wave, is trialled on the Isle of Wight. It relies on people downloading and using the app to be effective [NHS PROVIDERS 2020].

5 May 2020

The UK has the highest number of Covid-19 related deaths in Europe at 29,427 [NHS PROVIDERS 2020]. Sir Patrick Vallance tells the House of Commons Health Select Committee that earlier testing for Covid-19 would have been beneficial, but would not have prevented the spread of the virus [GALLAGHER, P 2020]. WHO announce 108 potential Covid-19 vaccines in development around the world, with eight approved for clinical trials [COHEN, E 2020].

7 May 2020

Baroness Dido Harding, Chair of NHS Improvement, is appointed to lead the UK government's test, track and trace programme [NHS PROVIDERS 2020].

9 May 2020

UK Transport Secretary Grant Shapps announces £2bn of investment to encourage walking and cycling, describing it as a 'once in a generation change' to the way the public travels [REID, C 2020].

The Big One

Sam Allen is an Infectious Diseases consultant in Ayrshire with over twenty-five years experience in managing outbreaks, including high consequence infectious diseases (Ebola, Lassa), and new and emerging infections (congenital Zika microcephaly, multi-drug-resistant TB and anthrax). In 2001, He was a first responder at Ground Zero in the immediate aftermath of 9/11, in which bioterrorism agents were suspected within the dust-cloud.

"This is the one that I had been waiting for. Like a big wave surfer, I had been waiting patiently for the next major global pandemic. At first, no one could be certain. Would the Chinese be able to contain it? Could we?

I have trained for sudden-onset emergent diseases and travelled to Sierra Leone and Brazil at the peak of their recent Ebola and Zika outbreaks. This time Mohammed didn't need to go to the mountain, for the mountain had come to Mohammed.

We were in the fortunate position of having had several test-runs for this pandemic, each bringing its own learning. In 2002, SARS-CoV-1 (Severe Acute Respiratory Syndrome, or SARS) rapidly disseminated across the globe through asymptomatic carriage on commercial flights. This first novel coronavirus could be quickly recognised (by the combination of acute respiratory symptoms and arrival from the disease epicentre in China) and persons affected could be isolated. The high case fatality (774 deaths from 8,096 cases) disproportionately affected front-line medical staff.

In 2009, the so-called swine flu, or influenza A H1N1, also spread with astonishing efficiency, affecting one in four of the world's population in two major waves a few months apart, but the case fatality rate was unexpectedly much lower (0.02 per cent). Ebola (2014) and Zika (2016) added to our learning but there would still be an 'unknown unknown' factor.

What marks SARS-CoV-2 (Covid-19) out as particularly malign is that it had found a sweet-spot for an infectious disease: an ability to transmit (via aerosol, droplet or fomites on surfaces) before a person showed symptoms, plus a human population lacking any immunity to this novel coronavirus.

Gladiators

The first wave arrived in Lombardy, northern Italy. 'Prepare for a tsunami' our Italian colleagues said. It was clear that the NHS capacity, with fewer ITU beds and ventilators per head of population than many of our European partners, could easily be overwhelmed. The early warning gave us three weeks to scale up. The response was monumental. It wasn't just China that could build a 1,000-bed hospital within a fortnight; Nightingale Hospitals rapidly sprang up across the UK, massively increasing bed capacity. Tens of thousands of volunteers signed up to support the NHS as retired doctors and nurses donned their badges and returned to work in their thousands to support frontline staff. Elective surgery was cancelled, and recovery rooms were repurposed to expand the number of ICU beds.

'Donning PPE for the first time in the ante-theatre feels like a gladiator in the Colosseum about to face the chariots of Scipio on the plains of Carthage', wrote my surgical colleague, Bob Meddings, drafted from an early retirement.

Life is Beautiful

Let's step back a moment to 2014. 'Life is beautiful.' Three words were all that the doctor could muster during his brief encounter in the Emergency Room to express his compassion towards a desperate, disconnected mother who had tried to end her life. She had been suffering from post-natal depression since giving birth nine weeks earlier. By her own admission she was not an easy patient. Words could not make her better. She wanted to die. Slowly, over six years

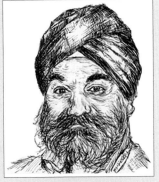

(*Portraits for PPE by artist Yaning Wu – Instagram @ portraitsforppe*)

she learnt to recover her meaning for living and remembered what the doctor had revealed to her. She had wanted to thank him and had tried to make contact but was unable. Data protection.

Today, fully recovered and now a trained counsellor, she recognised the doctor's image on the evening news, unmistakeable in his turban.

Dr Manjeet Singh Riyat, an eminent and highly respected Accident and Emergency consultant at Royal Derby Hospital featured on the front pages of every local paper. He had succumbed, at the age of 52, to coronavirus, during those early days of Covid-19. Like Dr Li Wenliang, the whistle-blower who raised the alarm in China, they are no less martyrs than the servicemen and women that we remember each Remembrance Day.

The R number
The coronavirus pandemic is the worst public health crisis for a generation and its control, as we learned from the daily No.10 briefings, is all about the R number. The basic reproduction number being the number of secondary cases for each positive case. Keep it below 1.0 and the epidemic will disappear; above 1.0 and numbers will increase exponentially. Stay at Home – Protect the NHS – Save Lives, in the new government tripartite vernacular, was all about lowering the curve. And it worked … for a while. The Swedish model (no restrictions, life as normal to hasten herd immunity) had been rejected by the scientific advisors, that is, the great and the good from SAGE (Scientific Advisory Group for Emergencies) and all that feed into them. But it wasn't just about the NHS. There was also the economy. Health versus Wealth. It is a complex equation as the two are inter-dependant. The No.10 Covid-19 Press Briefings reintroduced a politeness into the realm of politics that had been missing in preceding frenzy of Brexit. The statements, complete with PowerPoint graphs, and a poignant reminder that every life is precious, were as quintessentially British as a cup of tea. When before had we seen politicians routinely asking the questioner if they would like to come back on that?
    'Next slide please.'

No ordinary flu
Viruses cannot exist indefinitely in the environment. They require living cells from a human or animal host to exist and multiply. Coronavirus replicates very rapidly during early infection, producing trillions of virions capable of infecting the next person. The infective

period is relatively short, lasting 4–8 days for most, so lockdown will interrupt transmission.

On one level, Covid-19 is like any other flu-like illness and will inevitably join the host of circulating viruses that we have learnt to live with like seasonal flu. Four out of five people experience only mild or no symptoms, but for some it can cause severe respiratory illness leading to death from respiratory and multi-organ failure, the result of a 'cytokine storm'. The only positive is that the vast majority of children will have no symptoms, although they can still transmit the virus. Prospects of eradication lessen with news that Covid-19 variants have emerged in the mink population in Denmark and are probably circulating in domestic animals.

Covid-19 has thrown up fascinating para-phenomena: Covid fingers and toes, transient loss of smell (anosmia), multi-system hyper-inflammatory syndrome (previously described in children and associated with coronary artery aneurysms – Kawasaki syndrome) and long Covid syndrome.

Within days of the first clinical cases in the city of Wuhan, the genome for this novel coronavirus was sequenced and released to the scientific community. It was shown to be closely related to bat coronaviruses. What has followed is an explosion of research and development with Britain playing her part among a varied cast.

The geo-socio-political effects are no less audacious: the closure of borders to most world destinations, the furlough scheme, the 'eat out to help out' scheme, a billion of the world's children out of school, cancellation of school exams, the work-from-home revolution. Best of all was the housing of the homeless during lockdown.

Hedgehog
The effect of Covid-19 on humanity has been as dramatic as it has been cathartic. Here's Bob again: 'Covid-19 has stopped time. How often have you wished for time to stop and have a chance to 'regroup' and 'catch up' and start again? … The quietness, lack of cars, clear skies and exercising families are wonderful to see. The world is better for it. Time to press the reset button.'

For the first time in years, I saw a hedgehog.

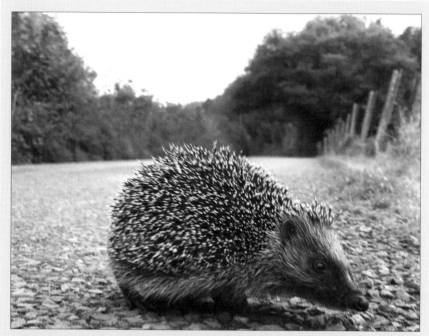

Life during lockdown. (*Alex Kumar Global Health Photography* ©)

The pause button has given us time out from the domestic maelstrom and professional inertia that steals the middle decades of life. In the introspection we have asked ourselves what is life for?

The new paradigm has affected almost every aspect of life – schools, education, healthcare, travel, business and the future economy. There are clearly beneficial effects for reducing emissions, though the tons of single-use plastics used as PPE is a singular cause of guilt.

The economic downturn has blighted the dreams and prospects of the young. I know of many seasoned NHS colleagues that have cried for the first time in years. Loss of control, the feeling of entrapment, futility, social isolation and loneliness has left many anxious for tomorrow. Not so the hedgehog, sparrows and their ilk. Perhaps this is nature reminding us collectively and individually that we are only visitors on planet Earth.

Covid-19 is likely to be with us for a long, long time. Smallpox apart, no other human infectious disease has been eradicated. But science will enable us to control it.

Keep breathing. Life really is beautiful."

Intensive Care Covid Diaries 6 – Dr Jenny Abthorpe

4 May 2020

Today I went to work. I sat on the train into London, watching the scenery rush past on a beautiful early spring morning. I pondered on the previous week's events when I had experienced a moment of real closure which started a slow healing process for me.

I had been on-call for ED, the outward facing bleep for ICU. Not much was happening there in the early morning so I was assisting the Outreach team. I was delegated to go and review a patient who had stepped down from ICU. He had a tracheostomy and needed a review as to whether it could be removed. To my delight, it was the patient I had intubated on the ICU almost a month to the day. The one I had urged to 'do well'. It was one of those moments that is meant to be.

I arrived on his ward and went to say hello. As I approached his bed, I felt a rush of emotion. He looked fantastic! He looked quizzically at me but smiled with equal delight as I explained who I was. I told him that it meant a lot for me to see him. I delivered the good news that I felt it was the right time to remove his tracheostomy. He was understandably nervous but after explanation and reassurance, I removed it.

Afterwards we chatted for a good while. He told me about his experience. His memories of his ICU stay (thankfully very little), his fears, his dreams for the future and his hope that he finally would make it home. He still refused to FaceTime or phone his son as he didn't want to get anyone's hopes up. But he had been texting. He said he would FaceTime the day he got home.

He was so grateful. We gave each other a hug. Both needing it as much as each other. And then I said goodbye and good luck. Leaving him in the care of his fantastic ward team. We had gone full circle and come out the other side.

Today it was business as usual. We have many patients doing well. Some are a bit static but there are some truly miraculous recoveries. Patients that have defied all odds. We still have new admissions coming in with Covid-19 but these are low numbers and we feel we know our adversary better now. The expanded ICUs are being decompressed and cleaned. Redeployed staff are being moved back into their base specialties … hopefully inspired by their brief stint in ICU. I could never have predicted the incredible collaboration, teamwork and solidarity displayed by all specialties towards our ICU team. Long may it continue. We are so grateful to all of them. True heroes.

Now it's time to try and focus on our own recovery. As the pace slows, emotions start to surface. Images of lines of ventilated patients are not easily forgotten. Nor the countless 'breaking bad news' phone calls. Or patients reviewed and intubated in ED. Or the losses. But the healing has begun.

My experience was mirrored up and down the UK, as the NHS reacted to an unprecedented challenge. The pandemic response by the NHS was immense and highly complex. A huge logistical challenge encompassing significant numbers of patients and their families, mobilising a large workforce, supplying vast amounts of PPE, medical equipment and drugs, rapidly expanding the number of ICU beds, training and educating re-deployed staff and implementing national research trials at short notice.

The NHS did not just cope, it saved thousands of lives. I will always be immensely proud of my profession and speciality in the part it played against Covid-19.

(This story first appeared in: *The NHS: The Story So Far*)

10 May 2020

The UK government updates its Covid-19 message from 'stay at home, protect the NHS, save lives' to 'stay alert, control the virus, save lives'. Leaders of the devolved governments decide to stick with the original slogan. A new alert scale is announced ranging from level one (green – Covid-19 is no longer present in the UK) to level five (red – Covid-19 epidemic is in general circulation and there is a risk of healthcare services being overwhelmed). The UKs Covid-19 recovery strategy to reopen society begins, with those who cannot work from home being encouraged to return to work the following day [NHS PROVIDERS 2020].

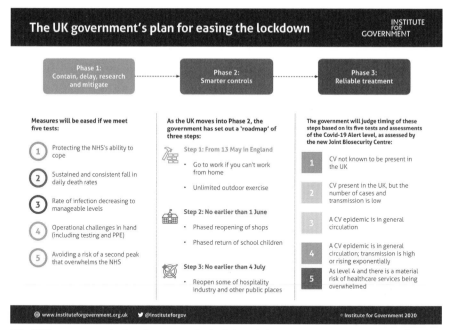

The UK government's plan for easing the lockdown'. (*Institute for Government 2020*)

11 May 2020

People in the UK are advised by the government to wear face coverings on public transport and in shops [NHS PROVIDERS 2020]. Teaching unions express concern at the government plan to reopen schools in June [LOVETT, S 2020].

12 May 2020

The UKs furlough scheme is extended until October. A quarter of the workforce, approximately 7.5 million people, are covered by the scheme, costing £14bn a month [NHS PROVIDERS 2020].

13 May 2020

Garden centres, sports courts and recycling centres reopen and unlimited exercise is permitted. House moves and viewings are also permitted under new coronavirus laws. Going on holiday, gatherings of three or more people from different household and visiting the houses of friends and family is still not permitted. In England, fines for breaching the rules are £100 for the first offence, up to a maximum of £3,200 [NPCC 2020].

14 May 2020
NHS England compile a breakdown of underlying health conditions among those who died of Covid-19 in hospital between 31 March and 12 May. One in four had diabetes. Other common conditions include dementia (18%), breathing problems (15%), chronic kidney disease (14%) and ischaemic heart disease (10%). Public Health England approve a blood test that can detect Covid-19 antibodies [NHS PROVIDERS 2020]. WHO's Director of emergencies Mike Ryan warns that Covid-19 may never go away [BFPG 2020].

15 May 2020
Matt Hancock announces that every resident and staff member in care homes throughout England will be tested for Covid-19 by early June. Between 28 December 2019 to 1 May 2020, 73,180 care home resident deaths occurred. This is 23,136 more than the same period a year earlier; 17.1 per cent of these deaths were due to Covid-19 (12,256) [NHS PROVIDERS 2020]. MPs are criticised for not prioritising care homes earlier in the pandemic [BBC 2020h], with cases of symptomatic people being discharged from hospitals to care homes to free up beds. Pandemic planning did not adequately consider care homes and many suffered with a lack of PPE. Notably, Brent Council had the lowest number of care home deaths in London likely due to them purchasing PPE for its care homes and creating a separate facility for any patient discharged from hospital [NHS PROVIDERS 2020].

18 May 2020
Anosmia – loss of smell and/or loss of taste is added to the official UK Covid-19 symptom list, meaning people experiencing this should self isolate along with their household. It is announced that anyone in the UK over the age of 5 with symptoms can now be tested for Covid-19 [NHS PROVIDERS 2020].

19 May 2020
Multiple security flaws are identified in the NHS Covid-19 tracing app and legislation is called for to prevent data being used for anything other than contact tracing. Over 21,000 contact tracers are recruited, including 7,500 healthcare professionals, all undergoing rigorous training to establish a test and trace operation by June. There has been no effective tracing in place in the UK since 12 March [NHS PROVIDERS 2020].

Symptoms triggering Covid testing

Testing for only the classic Covid symptoms of cough, fever and anosmia misses a significant proportion of positive cases. When NHS PCR testing was scarcely available at the start of the pandemic, restricting testing made sense. The ZOE Covid symptom study app examined data from 122,000 UK users who reported any potential Covid symptoms. The team identified users who reported a positive test and analysed their symptoms. They found that testing people with the classic triad picked up 69 per cent of symptomatic cases. If testing was expanded to people with seven key symptoms of cough, fever, anosmia, fatigue, headache, sore throat and diarrhoea, then 96 per cent of symptomatic cases would have been detected [ANTONELLI, M et al 2021].

Australia tested patients with any new upper respiratory symptoms from the start of the pandemic, advising:

If you have cold or flu like symptoms, such as a cough, fever, sore throat, shortness of breath or runny nose, even if these are mild, you should get tested for Covid-19 as soon as possible. People with mild symptoms can still spread the virus, and anyone with cold or flu-like symptoms should get tested.

Even those with symptoms of seasonal rhinitis (hayfever) were advised to undergo testing if there were any doubts they could have coronavirus – and Australia fared considerably better in this pandemic than the UK [AGHD 2020].

20 May 2020

The number of people in hospital in the UK with Covid-19 drops below 10,000 for the first time since March [NHS PROVIDERS 2020].

21 May 2020

No.10 announces that all NHS workers will be exempt from the immigration health surcharge that is usually applied to non-EU migrants to use the NHS. The charge is £400 per year (£624 from October 2020) [NHS PROVIDERS 2020]. Frontline staff, however, reported they were still being charged months later to access the very NHS for which they work and pay taxes. Groups such as the Doctors' Association UK lobbied for reimbursements of this charge for both staff and their dependents, and this was finally granted in October 2020 [DAUK 2020].

Organised Chaos

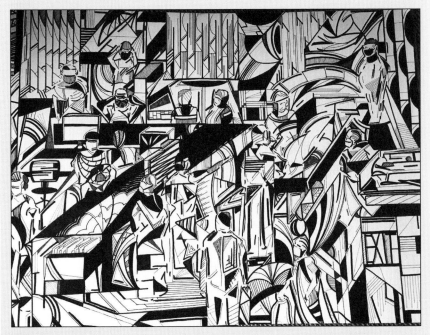

Organised Chaos.

Miss Sara Caterina O'Rourke is a Major Trauma Fellow in Edinburgh and the artist of the image 'Organised Chaos', an illustration of the Emergency Department at the height of the Pandemic's first wave.

I worked as second year foundation doctor (FY2) in the emergency department of the Royal Infirmary in Edinburgh during the pandemic. This is one of the busiest emergency departments in the UK. With training and rotations frozen amid the anxiety of the pandemic, I spent the best part of a year in the department. It became my home from home, my family and my social fix. Indeed, I considered myself lucky to be able to see other people at work.

In that time, I witnessed the department change. Everything became different – the staff were unrecognisable, our patient care forcibly emptied of much warmth due to our PPE camouflage. The department's physical fixtures – its equipment, layout and everyday customs were forced to comply with ever-changing regulations and we were constantly bathed in pools of sterilising chlorine. It was an organised chaos, a methodical yet somewhat dehumanising transformation.

For me, this picture depicts just that. It portrays the department during the pandemic – a microcosm of anxiety, unknowns and insurmountable pressures – somewhat hidden and depersonalised by aprons, gloves and masks. This picture was a gift for the department, for their support and their hard work – but also a testament that captured the experience shared by all of us there.

I wonder what it will be like to reinject colour into things again when this is all over.

NHS Covid Heroes?

Dr Michael FitzPatrick is a gastroenterology registrar and Co-Chair of the Royal College of Physicians trainees' committee. He discusses the widespread superhero rhetoric that swept through the UK during the pandemic, mainly on Thursday nights at 8pm.

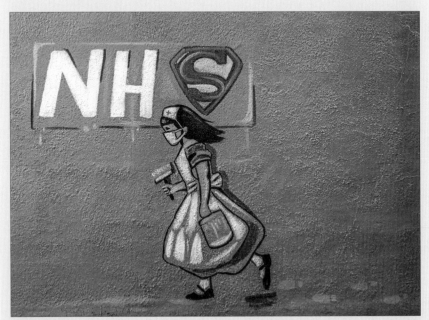

NHS Heroes. (*Mural by artist Rachel List at The Horse Vaults, Pontefract* (*instagram @ rachthepachel*))

Medical Royal Colleges attract a Hogarth-esque stereotype – pomp and ceremony, gold chains and portraits of dead white men, interminable committees and bursting wine cellars. I have been the co-chair of the trainees' committee at the Royal College of Physicians of London for a couple of years now, and the reality is very different. College leaders are jobbing consultants – practical, down to earth, and driven by a desire to improve our profession and the health of the nation. Although there probably are still too many old white men on the walls.

Our committee represents physicians in post-graduate training. Much of that work focuses on the training process – curricula, training programmes, post-graduate exams, and training quality – but we also act to ground the work of the college, and centre it on the reality of the world as junior doctors find it.

As Covid-19 spread, it was that second role that came to the fore. The committee became a de facto link between those leading the Royal College of Physicians, and the frontline experiences of junior doctors up and down the country. A usual workload of a few hours a week swelled to consume almost all our time, with everything on a tight deadline, often within hours. It was mentally and emotionally exhausting, but I am proud of the work we did to speak truth to power and get the viewpoint of front-line doctors heard.

This piece was written outside my RCP role, first on Twitter. It gained unexpected traction, and I ended up on Radio 4 reading a version of it for Inside Health. It was written back at the start of the pandemic, while the public still clapped, and politicians were lining up to laud healthcare workers. It is now August – and sadly, like Cassandra, the accurate predictions do not bring me joy.

We need to talk about heroes.
Doctors and nurses are not heroes. Calling them heroes (or saviours or angels) is well-meaning – a knee-jerk compliment born from gratitude and admiration during a time of crisis – but is ultimately both unhelpful and damaging. I also worry that this narrative is being co-opted, deliberately by some, to undermine the professionalism of the medical workforce, and silence their voice.

The Oxford English Dictionary tells us that a hero is 'a person who is admired or idealised for courage, outstanding achievements, or noble qualities'. From the Greek, the word was first used in those myths and legends about figures imbued with 'superhuman qualities and often semi-divine in origin'. In the ancient myths, heroes were nigh-on invincible. They battled against incredible odds and vanquished their enemies. Those same themes live on, in war movies, in comics, in the Marvel Cinematic Universe: Thor battling night elves, Captain America against Hydra, the Avengers against Thanos.

In these stories, many of these heroes are unpaid, rich volunteers. Thor is a King and a God, Tony Stark has more money than he knows what to do with, Batman is a rich recluse. They don't work to pay the bills, feed their kids, or pay off their medical school loans. They ARE their work.

These heroes, ancient and modern, are also semi-invulnerable. Bruce Wayne has his armour, Iron Man his suit, Captain America his vibranium shield. There are no personal protective equipment concerns here – these guys bring their own to the party. And when they die, they do so, well, heroically. It was their job, their inevitable lot, to die in battle. Think of Achilles and Patroclus in front of the walls of Troy, or Heimdall and Dr Strange in the fight against Thanos. Their heroism stemmed from their willingness to make the ultimate sacrifice. Heroes aren't scared, they don't baulk at personal risk.

How do we reward our heroes? Not with cash, that's for sure. We clap and cheer, we hold parades. We build statues and monuments, literally and metaphorically placing them on a pedestal, one which does not allow them to come down to the human level.

What keeps a hero going? Grit. Pluck. Inner strength. Moral fibre. They are better than us, stronger. They don't need appropriate working conditions, work-life balance, lunch breaks, or tea. They don't need duvet days or cat GIFs or psychotherapy. They are better than that. But if a hero is struggling psychologically, what do they do? How does Ironman deal with his post-traumatic stress and flashbacks following the battle for New York? How does Thor deal with his food binges and problematic drinking after Infinity War? By more work of course! More fighting! Bring me Mjölnir!

So, as we can see, heroes are almost entirely the wrong comparator with healthcare workers. But does this narrative, these clichéd metaphors in political speeches and newspaper headlines, matter?

Aren't the public, the politicians, the media, just being kind and supportive? I worry there's a darker side to this.

For there is something else that myth, comics, and cinema all tell us about heroes: they are only ever loved in the crisis. Batman goes back into hiding. Thor returns to Asgard. The heroes hide, they slink away. They're a threat now. No one wants to hear their thoughts on social inequalities or healthcare funding models. Back in your box.

The hero metaphor is therefore a useful tool for those who don't want to hear from doctors afterwards. Those in the 'Stay in your Lane' brigade, who don't want healthcare professionals to have a voice in our wider public and political discourse. Don't talk about PPE. Don't talk about student debt. Don't talk about public health or working conditions. Don't talk about healthcare funding.

Go back to the shadows.

This is very different if we reframe the narrative to one that centres around professionalism. For the views of professionals matter, both during the crisis, but importantly afterwards. They are not rewarded with medals, instead they need PPE, equipment, and training to carry out their roles. They don't work for claps and cheers on a Thursday evening, they work for remuneration commensurate with their expertise.

So that is why I know my colleagues are heroes. They are more than heroes, more real, more important, more valuable. They are highly trained, dedicated, caring professionals.

Thank you to all my colleagues who are working so hard in this pandemic. My heart goes out to the families of those professionals who have died, both here and abroad. Thank you for your work. Thank you for your service. And I hope a grateful society will listen to you after this.

22 May 2020

The UK Scientific Advisory Group for Emergencies publishes its evidence on the safety of reopening schools from 1 June and declare the risk very, very small, but not zero [GALLAGHER, J 2020].

26 May 2020
Matt Hancock announces at the daily briefing that there are now contracts in the UK to manufacture 2 billion items of PPE. Trials have commenced for selected NHS Covid-19 patients to be given anti-viral drug Remdesivir [NHS PROVIDERS 2020].

28 May 2020
The tenth and final 'Clap For Our Carers' takes place on doorsteps around the UK [WIKIPEDIA 2020c].

June

- 6,057,853 cases globally; 371,166 deaths
- 257,403 cases in the UK; 38,358 deaths
  (WHO 2020a, GOV.UK 2021)

Figure 1. Number of confirmed COVID-19 cases reported in the last seven days by country, territory or area, 26 May to 01 June**

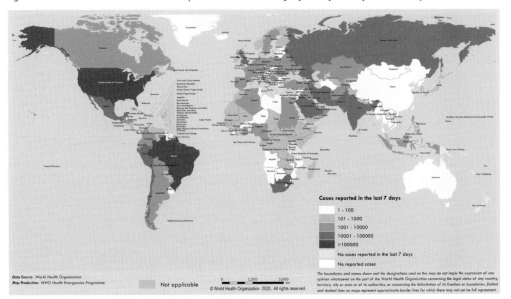

1 June 2020

The UK records the lowest increase in Covid-19 cases and deaths since lockdown started at the end of March. Lockdown rules are relaxed, and gatherings of people from more than one household are allowed, limited to six people outdoors [NHS PROVIDERS 2020].

2 June 2020

NHS Test and Trace eventually launches on 28 May to trace the contacts of anyone who tests positive for Covid-19. The daily briefing discusses the service, stating that anyone testing positive for coronavirus will be asked to share information about their recent interactions, including household members, and people with whom they have been in direct contact or within 2 metres for more than fifteen minutes. Contacts must stay at home for 14 days, even if asymptomatic, to stop unknowingly spreading the virus [NHS PROVIDERS 2020].

Pause

Dr Alexander Kumar is a global health physician, currently working as an Academic Clinical Fellow at King's College, London. He has been involved with infectious disease outbreaks across the world and volunteered in the setup of the London Nightingale hospital.

"Google defines the word 'pause' as 'a temporary stop in action or speech'.

As a child I remember having hand-me-downs in all too many forms, from clothing to music to ideas, from my elder brothers and sister. This included old VHS tapes, which required rewinding to watch a non-PG film, that I probably shouldn't have been watching in the first place. I always found the pause button an interesting concept. When I pressed it on the VHS player, there was a three or four stage triple clunk as the film ground to a halt a second or two later, creating a freeze-frame image with lines through it, leaving me to go and hunt down another Jaffa cake from the kitchen."

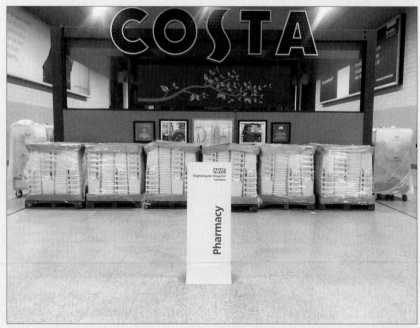

Costa Coffee in the London ExCel transformed into a pharmacy. (*Alex Kumar, Global Health Photography* ©)

Time flies

I have always been enthralled by the natural world and firmly believe there is no one on this planet who has seen it more than Sir David Attenborough. Decades have flown by, and in the past twenty years I've been lucky to have travelled the world and taken photos along the way to better understand this planet and its people. From tracking snow leopards in outer Mongolia to overwintering in Antarctica to pondering over the giant statues of a lost civilisation on a stopover on Easter Island. Medicine has been a passport for my boyhood curiosity, and my camera, a witness. I am now as used to hearing a shutter mechanism activate in a camera as I am counting heart beats through a stethoscope.

I've worked all over the developing world, as I often joke in my lectures … from Slough to Milton Keynes to Ghana to India. As a microcosm of the natural world an\d its wonders, I have always been interested in infectious and tropical diseases and their outbreaks and have managed to travel the world exploring them. I have tried not to be frightened but instead be led by my innate curiosity, combined with fact and preparation, when faced with potentially harmful infectious diseases.

In 2006 while still a medical student, I completed the first piece of HIV research in the Canadian Arctic, among Inuit. Every infectious disease is unique. Every outbreak is challenging in its own way – epidemics to pandemics, Afghanistan to Zimbabwe, from Anthrax to Zika.

My previous mentor, an infectious disease and arctic health specialist in Canada taught me that each pathogen is its own actor and displays its own theatrical story on its own stage, you just have to watch, study and recognise the play.

Infectious diseases threaten lives as they do security. Unusually for a doctor, global health security has also been an interest for me, and I have been lucky to have worked in this area for a number of years, though do not claim grand expertise. The global health security agenda focuses upon infectious disease outbreaks, but incorporates so much more from access to basic health care, education, food security and water scarcity – all fundamental determinants of health that perpetuate inequity and inequality.

Ebola virus

Ebola virus is unique and as equally fascinating as it is tragic. Causing one of the world's most fatal viral diseases, it is classified as a viral haemorrhagic fever, often leading to significant bleeding out of orifices before death. I had the opportunity to travel out to West Africa into the midst of the world's largest Ebola outbreak in history. After PPE and Ebola training in Geneva with Doctors without Borders, the world experts up until this outbreak, I completed a five-day training programme with the CDC in the USA. We were taught by staff who had first-hand stories of horror and death from the front lines.

I travelled via Liberia to Sierra Leone into the storm of another wave. On arriving at the Ebola Treatment Centre I gained my first insight to this blazing, tragic outbreak – a lady in her late twenties died in front of me, taking her last breaths alone, separated by a fence without PPE. I was unable to hold her hand.

The international press ran a circus. Ebola was ruthless as a virus – it took lives, maimed families and broke culture. Fortunately, with

Ebola, such an outbreak and perceived threat to the developing world, meant prevention and treatment was prioritised, and we now have several effective vaccines. Thanks to this sudden progress (we have known about Ebola since its discovery in 1976) we will never see such a large outbreak of it again. Rebuilding a country and health system after an Ebola outbreak could be seen as being easier than after a disease like Zika virus, which had its own disastrous effects – leaving thousands of affected children with disabilities requiring round the clock care and neurorehabilitation.

Zika virus
When I landed in North East Brazil, stepping off the plane at Recife onto the hot tarmac into the humid Atlantic breeze, I stumbled into a scientific mystery. How did this virus that originated in Zika (pronounced 'Zeh-kah') forest in Uganda end up causing microcephaly (small, mal-formed heads) in newborn babies in another country on the other side of the world? Transmitted by Aedes mosquitoes, it had swept through the Pacific islands causing another type of presentation altogether – Guillain-Barré syndrome – a medically notorious syndrome causing a recognisable ascending paralysis eventually stopping a person's chest and lungs from drawing in air.

I made several trips to Brazil, during its Zika epidemic. One trip allowed me to revisit certain units and families. I shall always remember one mother with her baby boy who was affected by Zika-microcephaly. Her partner had left her because of the burden of the disease on their child. She had her to mother help her, but the true burden of Zika virus was evident. Zika damaged society in a different way. It broke relationships and families and required more than a knee-jerk temporary response and one-off donation of funding, but careful planning and support into the future, long after it dropped off the media and political radars. After a disease dissipates, the impact from outbreaks, whether emotional or economic, remains and can span generations.

'Woo-hoo' virus
Let's be honest, the news media has cried wolf too many times regarding the threat of global pandemics. From swine flu to bird flu

outbreaks to rumoured killer bees – people stopped listening – the global public was too busy. But the real experts, (such as Professors Fauci and Farrar), who could decipher the hymn sheet, have always kept singing. Although no one could have predicted the scale and longevity of coronavirus.

As the first cases popped up in the UK in 2020, the doctors in a central London Emergency Department jovially continued on, sarcastically referring to this new underestimated threat as the 'Woo-hoo' virus. They remained in denial, underwhelmed, not grasping its threat or significance. Many of us did. This was long before countries succumbed to the enormous uncertainty, were forced to accept a new reality and were confronted by a lack of PPE, which was the only defence at the time against the possibility of ending up on a ventilator or worse.

Coronavirus cemented its place in history – from turning hearsay, 'the end is nigh' hypothesis, into real-life impact, suffering, loss and death. It went straight into the charts at Number 1, due to its devastating global cultural, human and economic impact. With regard to the hymn sheet – the monster the professors said and knew was coming, was born and released.

It was always going to come. The only question was where it would emerge from. As with Russian roulette, the natural world's virus-spawning revolver clicked round and round without discharge as the trigger was pulled, a handful of times in the past. We've been lucky, that's all. Until now. This time the viral gun went off.

But we have also been lucky with coronavirus. 'How so?', I hear you scream. It may sound crass or unthoughtful, and certainly comes with no disrespect to those who have been so severely impacted by this virus, but solely scientifically speaking we are actually very lucky to have had a virus with low-lethality and not another different virus or flu variant for example, that wouldn't have spared the young and whose overall mortality rate could easily hit 90 per cent across all age ranges. The natural world has proven itself more than capable in the past and for the way some of us have treated it, would have all the metaphysical reasoning to fight back against humanity. It is always a mistake to underestimate the natural world, infectious diseases and their outbreaks. The world learnt its lesson and has since ground to a standstill.

The great pause

I consider this time similar to the USA's great depression, a significant dent in culture and society. I will always refer to Covid and lockdown as 'the great pause' for this exceptionally unusual time. In life, a pause is often perceived to be an awkward sensation. Its unpleasant nature, characterised by its awkward silence, conjures anxiety. We struggle, pressured to speak but uncertain what to say next, confounded by what the future may hold. Like on the VHS player, this film of life has come to a sudden jolted-stop. We have all had to pause and to change and adapt the way we live, perhaps even forever.

NHS Nightingale Hospital London

'Unprecedented' became the buzz word to explain this great unknown, as coronavirus unfurled its veil on stage – we were, and still are, living in unprecedented times. When I first heard about London's NHS Nightingale hospital it sounded inconceivable, unimaginable and unbelievable. As the nation's biggest insurance policy against coronavirus and its consequences, money really didn't matter. NHS Nightingale was set up for the worst-case scenario, with the best intentions and sparing no necessity.

The press around it came in two distinct forms – those who appeared to understand its need and unfortunately, those who couldn't. A team like no other was formed from the Ministry of Defence, private building and supplier contractors, KPMG and NHS clinical and managerial staff expertly led by Barts Health NHS Trust. Everyone came together to orchestrate this remarkable feat – turning London's chosen venue – the Excel international convention centre – into what was planned to be the world's largest intensive care unit.

The Excel consists of two halls, the North and South event halls, with a total 939,649 square foot of column free space. It is massive. With 33ft high ceilings, noise reverberates around inside like water in a coconut. I entered the Excel and immediately recalled the last time I was there for an event where I got to interview the now deceased

Apollo 15 astronaut Al Worden for over an hour. The Guinness Book of Records recognises him as the world's most isolated human in history, having flown the farthest orbit from Earth around the moon, alone, while his two compatriots bounded around in moon boots below. His words rang truer than ever before. He spoke of orbiting the dark side of the moon and looking out from his porthole into the coldest, darkest universe of the blackest black, scared but in wonder, and was instead warmed by the greatest curtain of stars as bright as the eye could see. Aptly, it reminded me we must always find positivity, warmth and hope in times of strife, struggle and loss – something that has come natural to me. I squinted at the ceiling of the Excel, reimagining his loneliness and I thought to myself just how lonely these patients who come here will be if or when they do wake up. Before the sharp bat of reality beat me around the head. This wasn't a time to philosophise or romanticise, it was a time for a reality check. While this may well become the world's largest intensive care unit, with it arrives all the challenges and tragedy – it could easily have a mortality rate to match.

Inside as teams of construction workers, like ants, went to work, I was flabbergasted by the sheer scale of the project. Recalling images of the Spanish flu pandemic – stadiums or schools turned into large wards with the gaunt white angelic figures of nurses floating through alleviating the suffering and breathlessness.

Early in its conception, the Nightingale remained flat-pack, with ongoing pre-planning meetings. I was among around thirty clinical and managerial personnel with the challenge to put a working NHS service into a convention centre, with all the ethics, protocols, procedures, risk planning, governance and ultimately the care needed to treat it. The only caveat – it had to be safe and to be done as soon as would be physically possible.

I'd done table-top exercises for setting up health care in refugee camps in humanitarian crises, but this was another beast – unique in its set up – both an NHS hospital but chiefly a field hospital. A 2D flat-pack design event venue was to become a multi-thousand-bed cubicle ward. It was the busiest few weeks. The team swelled with expertise, with over 100 people present at the daily briefings. I was really a tiny and insignificant cog working alongside some large cogs, groups and mechanisms but tried my best. Each round table had its own team representing another piece of the puzzle to navigate a patient from being accepted, to the (outstanding) care they would receive, then onto what happened regarding their outcome – discharging home any survivors with appropriate and sensitive support for patients and families along the way.

The characters involved were proficient and effective. With enthusiasm and sensibility came hurdles including numerous politics and red tape. It had to be safe and it was. It is not my story to tell of the events or clinical cases which passed through London's NHS Nightingale hospital but what I would say is I was so impressed by the teamwork and comradery. Where one team member fell down and went off sick, another would pick up their pen and keep on writing. Witnessing the nursing team in particular at work, furthered and deepened my utmost respect and appreciation for this too often politically neglected profession.

Misinformation

Since coronavirus, there has been more misinformation spun out on social media and mainstream media than during any other event in history. The media and social media can be a poisoned chalice – it can be as powerfully constructive as it can be destructive. The stage has been set for coronavirus. These days it is all too easy to press a send button, whether it be to tweet, upload or post, without considering the dire consequences to public safety, by misunderstanding the information you are making or re-tweeting. Misinformation can be extremely harmful to health.

Doctor Andrew Wakefield was expunged from the UK medical system after his publication of an incorrect and fabricated link between the MMR vaccine and autism. This provided fuel to damaging and false campaign fires which anti-vaccinators still use to this day, despite such a link being entirely made up. Vaccines have saved hundreds of millions of lives, last year, this year and will do so into the future. Having worked in Bangladesh I was impressed to learn how vaccination has led to a decrease of 50 per cent in Bangladesh's mortality rate in under 5 year olds over the past decades. Children there are no longer dying of vaccine-preventable illness. This is the power of vaccination, substantiated by accurate study, statistics and facts.

We have a duty to remain factual and to educate ourselves with facts. Opinions matter but should never be mistaken for scientific fact – whatever the opinions are wrapped or dressed up in, underneath they remain only opinion.

One small step for man can be a giant leap for a virus

Viruses are inanimate. They don't crawl, move, fly or otherwise. They are essentially little syringes of DNA or RNA. They are incapable of replicating without a warm and welcoming host cell. We move them and we help them to replicate, allowing them to mutate. Similarly, as we move them, we can also stop them. We are all responsible for this. You don't always learn without experience or making your own mistakes. As doctors, we are required to measure risk against benefit in all facets of our work.

Scientific endeavour and innovation are hot on the heels of this virus, but we are always one step behind – we have to wait for concrete scientific conclusions from relentless and reliable studies before we conjure up a new vaccine against a new, emerging strain. It's an academic game of cat and mouse, where the mouse moves fast and mostly unpredictably. Our notoriously slow research protocols have had to adapt to keep up. However, at this time, and probably at any time in the future, vaccination is the only safe way out of this pandemic's global lockdown.

Infinite

In light of the significant challenges, we all face from climate change, overpopulation and coronavirus, you can only be impressed and reassured by the natural world. Whatever small and yet still insignificant footstep placed by humans on this 4.5-billion-year-old planet – since we have lived only for such a short blip our footprints have only sunk so deep. Coronavirus or no coronavirus, the natural world can hopefully right itself from our impact.

As with our first steps on the moon. We, together, as a human race can probably overcome any adversary. I hope we can find the path to success to see an end to unnecessary suffering and lockdowns, confinement within our four walls and Zoom cocktails.

Signposted by Neil Armstrong, I definitely do agree, 'if you're going through hell, keep going'.

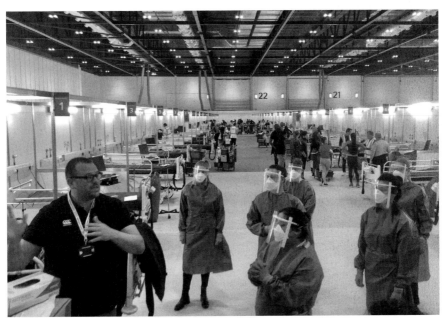

Dr Nick Murch, Acute medicine consultant seconded to the Nightingale to help induct and train a mixture of specialists and relative lay people. This was in the dummy ward area where we simulated a ward set up as part of the day zero sim project. Dr Murch worked alongside human factors and design experts including Bryn Baxendale, looking at the clinical areas for latent errors in the environment and testing procedures before opening. In-situ simulation also enabled further induction to the clinical environment. Feedback was it was the best induction many had had in their hospital careers (if they had ever had one). (*Alex Kumar, Global Health Photography* ©)

3 June 2020

The Prime Minister urges people with symptoms of Covid-19 to get tested. He also emphasises that gatherings should remain outdoors and not move inside as the risk of transmission is lower outdoors [NHS PROVIDERS 2020]. Black Lives Matter protests are held across the UK in solidarity with US anti-racist campaigners, following the murder of George Floyd on

25 May, who died in police custody after police officer Derek Chavin knelt on his neck for over nine minutes [HILL, E et al 2020].

8 June 2020
Passengers arriving to the UK by plane, train or ferry are required to self-isolate for 14 days in an attempt to keep case numbers down. Countries such as New Zealand have had quarantine measures in place since the start of the pandemic. WHO said in February that measures which significantly interfere with international travel may only be justified at the beginning of an outbreak [SKY NEWS 2020].

9 June 2020
Globally, the number of Covid-19 cases reaches 7 million. New Zealand has reported no new infections for two weeks, while in the UK, the lowest daily death toll since 22 March is recorded of fifty-five deaths [BFPG 2020]. Thirty medical organisations write to the government raising concerns at the finding that black, Asian and ethnic minority people are twice as likely to die from Covid-19 [HASAN, R 2020].

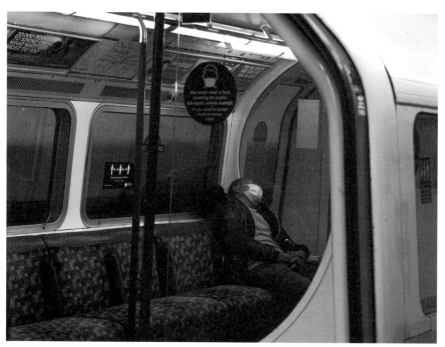

A masked traveller on the Bakerloo line, London, 2020. (*Photo by john crozier on Unsplash*)

10 June 2020

Professor Neil Ferguson, the government scientist whose advice was crucial in persuading the government to implement the lockdown measures, says that half of the lives lost to Covid-19 could have been saved if the measures had been introduced a week earlier [BBC 2020i].

15 June 2020

Shops and outdoor venues such as farms and zoos reopen. Wearing a face covering on public transport becomes mandatory [NHS PROVIDERS 2020].

16 June 2020

Trials find that dexamethasone (a cheap and widely available steroid medication) can reduce mortality among critically ill hospitalised Covid-19 patients [NHS PROVIDERS 2020]. Footballer Marcus Rashford launches a campaign to end food poverty, motivated by the children who were going without their free school meals during lockdown. His open letter prompted the government to continue meal vouchers during the school holidays, an initiative they had originally argued against [PIDD, H 2020].

19 June 2020

The UK's chief medical officers downgrade the coronavirus alert level from four to three following a steady decrease in cases [NHS PROVIDERS 2020].

23 June 2020

Health leaders write an open letter in the BMJ calling for the government to launch an urgent review to determine whether the UK is prepared for a second wave of Covid-19 [ADEBOWALE, V ET AL 2020]. Meanwhile in Brazil, trials of the Oxford AstraZeneca Covid-19 vaccine begin [BFPG 2020].

26 June 2020

The quarantine regulations are changed to allow people to holiday in places such as Spain and Greece without being obliged to quarantine for 14 days on their return [BFPG 2020]. This follows the declaration of a 'major incident' the day before when beaches on the south coast of England are overwhelmed with sun seekers [BBC 2020j].

Call the Midwife

Anna Startup is a midwife at the Cumberland Infirmary in Carlisle, where she continued to work throughout the pandemic.

First Wave

"I don't think the pandemic hit maternity services as hard as we feared it might when the virus first broke out in the UK. I was most concerned when I heard that extra hospital beds were being installed in our local leisure centre and that the army would be assisting. We knew that our work to support women and their families would carry on regardless, but there were a lot of people feeling anxious, not least the pregnant women.

I work in a small consultant led unit and during the first wave I only cared for two women with symptoms of Covid-19 and a handful of others who tested positive but had no physical symptoms. It took us a while to figure out what PPE was needed and how to organise our wards in case of an influx of pregnant women needing single rooms. A little like the UK government's response, our practice changed gradually. Daily updates came from Public Health England, the Royal Colleges and our hospital Trust. Returning to work after being off-duty for a day or two felt challenging to keep up with the latest advice.

To begin with we did not have enough masks to allow for frequent changing, we were unsure how long each box was going to need to last and how many more boxes we would receive. Looking back, the media headlines probably made that feel worse than it actually was, but we weren't to know that at the time. There were so many considerations: can we safely allow birth partners or visitors in the unit? Should we change our masks after each patient, each shift or every time we left the room, or every twenty minutes (in case the moisture made it less effective)? We were trained in the correct way of donning and doffing the protective wear and disposing of it safely. We spent some time practising this as we realised that we would need to be quick when responding to emergencies. In fact, the call bells have never sounded for so long because of the time it takes to get the gear on! Then we have had the issue of how to manage theatre cases (where a general anaesthetic is considered high risk in terms of Covid-19), particularly when the woman's status was unknown. How could we protect patients and staff in this high-risk area when often the theatre teams would be caring for Covid-19 positive people elsewhere in the hospital? Despite our own worries and personal discomfort from wearing PPE, staff pulled together to do the best job possible and the thanks, love and praise of the nation has been overwhelming.

Midwives and doctors in my unit noticed far fewer women telephoning with minor issues, the unit was much quieter for several weeks with barely any triage cases to see. This effect has yet to be audited in terms of rates of morbidity or missed problems in pregnancy of course. The only women who wanted to attend were those in labour or who had no other choice. There were no triage appointments for light or vague reasons, I think people were genuinely staying away to be safe. I believe that this effective shielding by pregnant women protected both them and us. Once restrictions relaxed, we saw an increased volume of triage cases (particularly as face-to-face GP appointments were probably a little harder to get) with the main problem being mental health issues. Women who had kept it together and stayed home for weeks now started to present with mental health symptoms triggered by less social contact, with the ensuing lack of sleep. Unfortunately, there was also a rise in domestic abuse and child safeguarding concerns since people were confined to small spaces together with the worries around jobs and money.

Things remain tough for pregnant women and their partners. All those long dreamed-of birth plans have been abruptly squashed. Women can only have one birth partner with them when in established labour and once they are in the single birth room, they are encouraged to stay put rather than pop in and out. This presents some logistical issues for them usually, including having to sleep on a chair, not always having regular meals if they are the birth partner and not being able to pop home to sort out pets or similar. To begin with everyone was very understanding about this. Now that restrictions are being lifted staff face the frustrations of families still denied access to the mothers and the new babies if they need to stay in hospital. Grandparents and others who were previously trying to stay home are being asked to help with children for days at a time.

Women can only use a birth pool if confirmed Covid-19 negative. There is no home birth service as we prepare for staff shortages if cases run high. I have heard about two formal complaints, one regarding the fact that we did not allow a father in to watch the antenatal scan and one because the home birth service was suspended. I'm sure there will be more. No visitors are allowed in to provide support or cuddles, it's so disappointing for people.

Interestingly, it's not all bad news. The restrictions have brought some benefits apart from reducing the spread of the virus. The fact that we are seeing fewer babies with a concerning weight loss at day five and ten after birth has made us realise how many interruptions to feeding new mothers are typically faced with in the postnatal period. Covid-19 advice has perhaps led to more privacy and rest during that baby-moon period, leaving nature to work its wonders. The other really noticeable change for us on the maternity ward was that we stopped having to put down what we were doing to answer the door or let visitors out all shift – selfish perhaps, but a much calmer, less stressful environment."

Second Wave – January 2021
"Since I last wrote my thoughts about how maternity services have been affected during the Covid-19 pandemic things have changed. We are almost a year on with no let up, and the situation during what we are calling the second wave is far worse. New, more virulent strains combined with a jaded public less inclined to follow social distancing rules have led to weekly cases being seen in my unit. I saw less than five patients with Covid-19 positive swab results in the first wave, but I have several each week at the moment.

Thankfully, it is still the case that not many of our pregnant women are very ill with symptoms, but we swab all admissions now, so regularly see how widely spread the virus has become. Sadly, I know we have also had some maternal deaths in our area, and we are now quite used to hearing that staff members, or members of their families, have been taken by the virus too. I have found it very depressing to hear how much strain my colleagues in the rest of the hospital have been under. I don't suppose anyone knows the statistics yet but it feels like, if they aren't dealing with Covid-19 patients they are increasingly seeing suicide attempts and issues arising from poor mental health. The hospital has been needing to transfer patients out for care and struggling to manage the day-to-day staffing and capacity issues that were trying enough before the pandemic started.

In the midst of the second wave, we have experienced an increase in requests for home births. I fear this has arisen from women feeling anxious about coming into hospital for care or difficulties in arranging childcare for older siblings. It has become challenging to staff our unit at times and we have often had to use the midwives who were on-call for home births to staff the labour ward to cover the staff who are off sick or having to self-isolate. We don't use any agency staff, so midwives have needed to be flexible, work extra and change shifts at short notice. Our hospital Trust asked us to postpone our annual leave to help the staffing crisis, so fatigue is setting in.

The pandemic has a knock-on effect for the whole NHS. We are having to explain to women requesting home births that realistically the ambulance service may be slower than usual and that if we cannot spare midwives to come out to them, they would have to either come into hospital to give birth or take responsibility for birthing alone. I know this has caused everyone concerned a lot of anxiety. We all surely look forward to better times.

The vaccine has been eagerly accepted by staff and as far as I see they are rolling it out very effectively where I work. We have been asked to wait a little longer for the second dose, but it brings us some hope and light at the end of the tunnel."

30 June 2020
The entertainment industry suffers a further blow, learning that theatres will remain closed until at least January 2021. The WHO declares that this pandemic is far from over [BFPG 2020].

The NHS is in Crisis

Dr Neil Barnard is dual trained in intensive care and emergency medicine and currently works as an emergency medicine consultant in the Midlands. He is a South African medical graduate and has recently lived and worked in New Zealand.

"The events of 2020, in which a new and unforeseen respiratory pathogen plunged the world into crisis, hit the NHS especially hard. The UK has suffered one of the worst death tolls in the world. Given that the results of the Cygnus report from 2016 [PHE 2016] were largely ignored, it is disingenuous to suggest that the UK could not have prepared for a crisis of this nature. It is also true that even if the government had had the political will to prepare adequately, the NHS has been left woefully under-resourced to deal with this pandemic.

Winter crises in the NHS are not a new phenomenon. Every year, without fail for the last ten years of my working life within the NHS, the organisation has lurched from one winter crisis to the next. Frightening statistics of bed shortages, ambulance waits and 'care' being delivered in corridors are splashed across the newspapers annually. The cause is almost always an influenza-like respiratory virus and it is mostly the frail and elderly people in our population who are disproportionately affected.

This time, the virus has a name and a face. This time, we are counting these statistics in a daily macabre ritual of learned scientists exhorting us all to 'do our bit' as the death tolls continue to rise. As with many aspects of our lives during the current pandemic, SARS-COV2 has not broken our healthcare system but has rather exposed the pre-existing cracks within it. Similar to the married couple during lockdown who have realised that they can't bear to spend so much time together, the Covid-19 crisis has laid bare the structural inadequacies of the NHS.

The NHS is frequently held up as a symbol of how great Britain can be. It was the centrepiece of the Olympic games opening ceremony in 2012 – that great tribute to all things British. Many of my colleagues speak in gushing terms of how proud they are to work for it. I can't honestly say the same thing and I must confess, although it is heresy to do so, that I have no great love for the NHS. Don't misunderstand me. As a concept, I am absolutely supportive of the system. The aim of universal access to health, free at the point of use and funded by proportionate contributions of the population is a noble and just one. Health is an inalienable human right. I am not, however, proud of the NHS as an organisation. Covid-19 has laid bare the organisational failings of the NHS. The blame for these failings must be laid squarely at the door of the successive governments responsible for the decisions which drive the health service.

Since the global financial crisis, the policy of the ruling Tory party in the UK has been one of financial austerity. In the midst of all of this, the party line was that NHS funding would be ring-fenced or even improved. Sure enough, since 2015, the NHS budget has increased by 1.6 per cent a year. What is perhaps little known is that with the ever-increasing cost of healthcare and the challenges presented by an ageing population, in order to merely maintain services at current levels, budget increases of at least 3.4 per cent per year are required. If the recommendations of the NHS long term plan are to be realised, the annual increases required are 4.1 per cent or £4bn [CHARLES, A et al 2019]. Since the wage budget is one of the largest components of NHS spending, it is obvious that this has been a target for the 'efficiency savings' NHS managers have been required to make.

The staffing crisis in the NHS has been well documented. According to NHS digital, in June 2020 the NHS had a shortfall of 84,000 FTE staff [NHS DIGITAL 2020]. The pandemic has only intensified this problem, and in November 2020, a further 82,000 NHS staff were recorded as absent from work with 42 per cent of these linked to coronavirus [LINTERN, S 2020]. This figure included almost 27,000 nurses and 4,000 doctors – not to mention all of the allied health workers like physiotherapists or laboratory scientists and radiographers who keep our lab and X-ray facilities functioning.

It is little wonder that there are fewer and fewer staff available. Since 2010, wages for NHS staff have not kept pace with inflation, with senior doctors seeing a real terms pay cut of 14 per cent [DAYAN,M 2020]. Nursing bursaries were scrapped in 2017 only to be reinstated for September 2020 when numbers of nursing applicants fell dramatically [CAMPBELL, D 2019]. A starting salary for a degree trained nurse is currently £24,907 per year [CARMICHAEL, C 2021] in a profession which is dominated by women who often take on multiple caring roles outside of work and are more likely to work part-time. Compare that with the ALDI shopping chain graduate program which offers a £44,000 starting salary and a BMW 3-Series [ALDI 2021].

The greatest asset the NHS has is it's people and I am overwhelmed on a daily basis by the people I work with. Almost every NHS staff member I have ever met, whatever their role, has invariably been of outstanding character. This dedicated workforce, especially those on the frontline, will almost always prioritise the health of their patients over their own. I have forced junior doctors to go home after they have worked additional hours without pay; I have seen nurses jump in to help with a crisis as they have been leaving and I have been amazed at how many staff will ignore their own health to come in to work when they are not feeling well because 'the department needs me'.

The sort of people who tend to work for the NHS are, on the whole, not motivated by money and are selfless people working hard to make a difference in a demanding and stressful environment because they genuinely care. It is an immutable fact that when staff numbers are low, patient care suffers. There is a powerful force in the NHS which is difficult to quantify but is vital for the functioning of the service. This is the goodwill bank. Overstretched staff are frequently found working extra hours, going the extra mile or mucking-in to help out. This is done without the expectation of being paid. NHS staff just care. Leaving work on time when a patient needs help and there is nobody else to provide it, is simply not the done thing. The NHS has relied on this goodwill bank for years to keep the service running, and right now, it is running dangerously low on capital. Staff are leaving the NHS in droves [CAMPBELL, D 2020] and those that remain face increasing levels of burnout or compassion fatigue [RIMMER, A 2020].

Years of pay cuts, changes to terms and conditions and the strain of covering shortfalls in rotas have left staff less willing to muck-in and far more likely to work to rule, treating the health service more as a job than as the vocation it is often purported to be. The language of vocation was heard during the first wave of the pandemic when NHS staff were called 'heroes'. It makes a good sound bite when politicians call us heroes, but our expectations of a hero is that they sacrifice themselves for the greater good. Thrust into the breach without adequate provision of PPE, it is unsurprising that care staff have the second highest risk of death from Covid-19 by occupation [ONS 2021]. They were thrown into Covid-19 wards with little more than flimsy aprons and surgical masks to protect themselves. Subsequent evidence has revealed what we all knew – this was woefully inadequate.

Throughout the Covid-19 crisis, we have repeatedly heard how the NHS is running at capacity and is working flat-out to increase this. Capacity is a function of staff numbers and of beds. The concept of an NHS bed is a curious one. While the layperson might simply think that a bed is a metal structure with a mattress and some bedding, the bed is in fact a unit of care and has various requirements depending on its location. Determining adequate nursing ratios is a complex business and is dependent not merely on the number of patients, but how unwell each patient is. Patients with greater numbers of co-morbidities that we hear about so much with Covid-19 reporting are invariably more complicated to manage and the skill mix of the staff greatly determines what level of care can be provided. Even the patient requiring the least complicated level of hospital care (usually a frail elderly person who has limited medical need but is in the hospital for social reasons) requires that bed to come with a nurse to provide medications, an HCA to help with basic care, a cleaner to ensure hygienic conditions and a myriad of support staff to complete the mountain of paperwork that is attached to NHS care. At the other end of the scale is the critical care bed, where each individual patient requires all of the above, plus round the clock support from a highly trained specialist nurse as well as input from medical staff who are responsible for the majority of clinical decision making.

Despite an increasingly ageing population in the UK, with their increased care requirements – NHS beds have been consistently reduced over the last ten years [EWBANK, L et al 2020]. The pandemic has highlighted the short-sightedness of these cuts. As Covid-19 emerged, hospitals were split into red and green (clean/ dirty) zones to prevent cross-contamination. The reconfiguration of bed spaces and the increased complexity of admitted Covid-19 cases has led to a reduction in the capacity of NHS trusts to admit patients. This capacity is based on physical space, staffing numbers and patient acuity. Entire hospitals have been reconfigured to maintain distance between beds, which has led to a further decrease in capacity. So, although there have been statistics in the press showing that fewer people have been admitted to hospital for all causes over 2020/21, this should be interpreted in context. Fewer attendances have been offset by a far greater proportion of beds lost. Any 'spare' capacity created has been as a result of cutting or cancelling elective services and redeploying the staff working in these areas to other acute care units. This has in turn led to the longest waiting lists in NHS history [LINTERN, S 2021], and delays in cancer diagnosis [GEDDES, L 2020]. The British Medical Association offers a grim analysis of how long it will take us to recover from the impact of Covid-19 – and this was even before the introduction of the latest winter lockdown [BMA 2020].

The most important question for the future therefore is: 'What does the public want from the NHS and how much they are willing to pay to get it?' The NHS is not in a position to pay for all treatments regardless of cost. It is for this reason that the National Institute for Health and Care Excellence (NICE) makes value judgements about treatment based on quality adjusted life years (QALY). A QALY refers to a unit of healthy life. Any treatment which is likely to be approved by NICE will cost £20,000 – £30,000 per QALY gained. Some treatments, like vaccination, provide long term quality of life at minimal cost, whereas some cancer treatments will cost a great deal of money with little difference in overall QALYs gained.

While we hate to talk of rationing of care, the pandemic has again brought the inadequacies of the NHS into sharp focus. Medical staff have had to make daily decisions as to who would benefit most from precious intensive care beds and high-level intervention. The flip side of that coin is that we have also been deciding which patients are unlikely to benefit from that level of care and therefore have a 'ceiling of care' put in place, beyond which further intervention leads to greater harm than good and is not in the patients' best interests.

The question is not *if* we'll face another pandemic but rather *when*. As humans are living in greater proximity to each other and we encroach on the habitats of animals, the opportunity for crossover of viruses from animal species to humans is ever greater. In order to prepare appropriately for the next event, we need to learn the lessons from this pandemic. Much has been written about the decisions taken by this government which have led to the UK having the greatest death toll in Europe and the fourth highest in the world. The science of lockdowns isn't a settled one and indeed, the World Health Organisation does not recommend them as a primary response to a pandemic. The long-term effects of lockdown may indeed cause more death than has been prevented. No doubt all of this will be debated in time and will inevitably be discussed in lengthy and drawn out independent enquiries.

My experience of recent travel to New Zealand certainly shows some of the potential benefits of an early and aggressive lockdown. After arriving in New Zealand, I was directed by bus to a hotel where I was forced to remain for two weeks without visitors. I endured two Covid-19 PCR tests and only after both of these returned negative results, was I allowed outside. At that point, the difference in life was immediately apparent. It was, in a word, normal. I was able to see friends, hug them and go with them to pubs and sporting events. When I worked in emergency departments in New Zealand, there were no red or green areas, no masks getting in the way of communication with patients and no lengthy ambulance waits before patients could be offloaded into the departments for definitive care.

The challenge for New Zealand going forward will be how it manages the reopening of the country. Without a significant vaccination policy and ongoing strict border controls, New Zealanders, for the last year naive to the coronavirus, will inevitably be exposed, which will lead to community cases and disease. The alternative is for the country to remain locked down for many more years until the rest of the world is adequately vaccinated.

Regardless of whether the correct response will be proven to be the Swedish herd immunity approach or the New Zealand 'zero Covid' method, it is clear that the UK has succeeded in neither of these strategies and has instead flip-flopped between the two, blighted by poor communication and inconsistent leadership. The UK has a population at risk from severe Covid-19 and it is the result of our healthcare system that we have a population that is elderly but not necessarily healthy. Risk factors for severe Covid-19 apart from age include chronic disease like obesity, diabetes and chronic lung disease. Environmental factors such as Vitamin D deficiency play a role too. In order to be prepared for the next pandemic, not only must we learn the lessons of policy failures, but we must prepare the population to be resilient to the effects of any new virus. This would involve an emphasis on healthy weight management, Vitamin D supplementation and addressing the systemic inequalities which have led to the BAME community shouldering the majority burden of these chronic lifestyle diseases.

We need a mature debate about how best to care for our elderly and infirm population who will just as easily be harmed as benefited by hospital admission at the end of their lives. It is time for our leaders to truly follow the science and encourage discourse as opposed to the politicking that has characterised the Covid-19 debate thus far."

July

- 10,357,662 cases globally; 508,055 deaths
- 284,914 cases in the UK; 40,766 deaths
  (WHO 2020a, GOV.UK 2021)

Figure 1. Number of confirmed COVID-19 cases reported in the last seven days by country, territory or area, 25 June to 1 July **

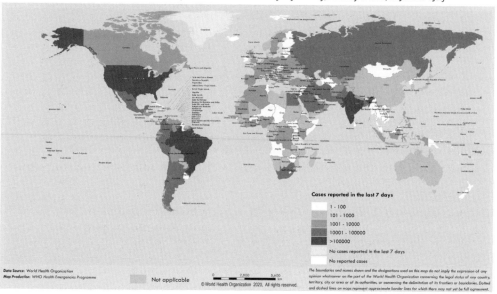

3 July 2020

The government announces a list of countries where English tourists can visit without self-isolating on their return. These changes do not apply to the devolved Nations where quarantine restrictions apply for all arrivals outside of the UK. According to a UN report, global tourism is expected to lose £3.3tn due to the pandemic [BFPG 2020].

4 July 2020

Lockdown restrictions are relaxed across England as pubs, restaurants, barbers and places of worship reopen to the public. The city of Leicester is excluded from the relaxations due to its high numbers of Covid-19 cases [BBC 2020k].

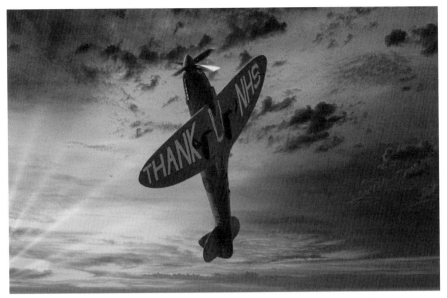

(Brendy Esler. Photo taken over Antrim Area Hospital as a 'thank you' to the NHS)

5 July 2020

The NHS celebrates its 72nd birthday with a national round of applause and a Supermarine Spitfire fly-past over several hospitals in the South of England.

Being a New GP Partner during a Pandemic – Rural

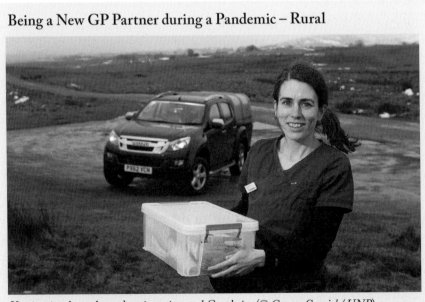

Vaccinating housebound patients in rural Cumbria. (© *George Carrick/UNP*)

Dr Rose Singleton is a GP Partner at a rural Practice in Cumbria. She took on this challenging new role only a few months before the pandemic hit and shares her experiences of dealing with this.

"At some point in early 2019 I had an epiphany – or was it a crisis? I wasn't happy in my job as a salaried GP. I liked the patients and my colleagues, but I thought the system could be better. My small voice was politely listened to, but it didn't carry much heft and I was starting to feel frustrated with just doing what I was told. I had ideas to make things better and more efficient, I wanted to improve care for patients and help shape the practice agenda. My opportunity came in the form of a 'salaried with a view to partnership' vacancy in a small rural practice. After a successful application and six months as a salaried GP I transitioned to my role as a GP partner on the 1 January 2020.

Becoming a partner meant I joined a team of four other GPs. As business owners and independent contractors for the NHS, partners are ultimately responsible for the practice; employing staff to carry out NHS work to our list of around 4,400 patients and shaping the environment in which that happens. I bought into the business and became self-employed. The pay was generally better, but the responsibility was huge. Managing staff, a building, finances, self-employment and everything else that running a business involves – albeit with the help of a practice manager – is a big addition to the clinical workload of a GP, so partnership isn't for everyone. In some ways I hadn't wanted it to be for me. I'd never seen myself running a business; I wasn't sure I had the right skills and I was worried about the extra stress it might involve but I couldn't shake the nagging voice in my head, spurring me to put my ideas into action.

The impact of coronavirus has come hand-in-hand with my journey as a new partner. It has been all-consuming and in parts, incredibly stressful, with everything that was hitherto considered standard practice being redefined through the prism of Covid-19 and its associated restrictions. Our role as partners was not just to oversee the changes and shepherd our staff and patients through it, but to be on the ground and get stuck in the sticky quagmire of the 'new normal', once we'd figured out what that even was.

Government guidance was Kafkaesque in its illogicality and nightmarish complexity, and often subject to change without warning. Vital information was buried in a rabbit hole of hyperlinks sent through on emails which led onto increasingly complicated documents, sometimes hundreds of pages long. I felt a new solidarity with other industries, leaders and business owners who were trying to navigate this seemingly impossible new territory. Interestingly, the experience felt familiar to a number of patients and staff in our rural farming community, who were reminded of the regulations imposed during the foot-and-mouth outbreak of spring 2001.

Vast changes were made in our surgery: alterations to the structure of the building; the working practices of staff; an overhaul of how patients accessed their care and even how we looked, dressed and behaved as clinicians. For all of us, it was vital that we carefully balanced Covid-19 restrictions with providing high quality, responsive care. The benefit of being a small group of partners meant we didn't have impenetrable layers of management to navigate in order to change something. Our locus of control was consistently close to the action, and we could quickly respond to feedback and make changes and improvements as needed. It was great to be so responsive, but sometimes it felt overwhelming, and I wish my brain could have been fitted with a quantum chip to process it all.

Becoming a partner has also changed my identity as a doctor. As a salaried GP and junior doctor before that, I could lament indulgently about problems that I knew I couldn't do anything about and collude with patients when they raged about the system. While my new role has little impact on national or regional health policy, what matters to many patients and staff in our little surgery is affected hugely by decisions made by the partners, meaning there is no more hiding away from critical feedback – and that can be anything from how long it takes to see a nurse, to stocking the wrong biscuits in the tea room. I've gained the ability to make a difference, but I must also shoulder the burden of responsibility for bad decisions and live with the consequences of the challenging ones.

Alongside forging my new identity as a partner, the impact of Covid-19 has simultaneously resulted in the loss of a different part of my GP identity. Changes to the building mean I no longer have my own room and most consultations now take place on the phone. I have been wearing scrubs to work rather than my own clothes and we have been using PPE in the form of mask, apron and gloves for every face-to-face patient interaction. At a time when I should be developing what could be lifelong relationships with patients, it feels instead like I have morphed into 'generic doctor' on the phone or in her 'generic consulting room'. My vision of the caring and empathic GP partner in a homely rural surgery has been uprooted and transplanted with an imposter who looks and feels a lot more like an efficient yet transient junior doctor in the Emergency Department.

Consultations have often felt more transactional than therapeutic, eroded by both physical and psychological barriers to good communication, and the feeling that Covid-19 is fraying the edges of the delicate doctor-patient relationship. It's an ironic juxtaposition, that at a time when I've reached what should be a high point in my career, my job has been stripped of many of the aspects of personalised and family-orientated medicine that made it such an attractive prospect in the first place.

Going back to 2019 – was it an epiphany or a crisis? From some perspectives, my timing looks terrible: taking on a huge new responsibility that coincides with one of the biggest crises the NHS has ever faced. There have been times when I have wondered why on earth I took this on and if, with the benefit of foresight, I would have turned my back and continued plodding along in my salaried role? I've thought about it, and I think I would still make the same decision. If I'd stayed in my old job, I can only imagine the frustration I would have felt about the double whammy of Covid-19 disrupting everything yet not having agency to do anything about it. The coronavirus pandemic has been a demonstration of the exact reasons I wanted to become a partner in the first place; to have some control and influence where I felt it mattered. The highs and lows of partnership have come thick and fast, but my plunge in at the deep end has accelerated my development as a leader, manager and decision maker, hopefully leaving me better prepared to face the challenges of the future.

Looking ahead, as the impact of coronavirus wanes, our group of partners can make our own decisions about what we do in that future, taking some of the positive changes forwards and banishing the most challenging. Importantly for me, I know that as the business evolves and adapts, my voice will be heard, and although I may currently look like a generic doctor, at least I know I won't be treated like one."

Being a New GP Partner during a Pandemic – Urban
Dr Charlotte Gooding is a GP Partner in the North-East of England.

As a new GP partner, dealing with a pandemic was my first big challenge. As things started to ramp up, I realised that we needed to firstly protect patients and staff from the disease. We had already started to put signs up around the surgery in early March, telling people not to enter the premises if they had travelled from any of the Covid-19 affected areas. We disconnected our touch screen booking system. At this point, we were criticised for being overly cautious, but now I'm glad we had already started making plans, as it seemed that literally overnight, things escalated and we had to completely overhaul our way of working.

Perspex screens were put up; doors were closed and a door entry system installed so that we could check each person entering the surgery. Our admin teams were split into two teams to limit the number of staff in the building at one time. Waiting rooms were marked out at strict 2m distancing of chairs and we got into the habit of cleaning everything in our consulting rooms on a regular basis through the day.

As a GP, I love to see my patients, and I have strong relationships with many of them. To transition to a total telephone triage system was a huge shock and felt contrary to everything I love about my role. It was very sad. Our job relies on our connection and communication skills with patients and it felt like barriers were being placed in the way of this. I was also very scared – worried how I could protect myself and my family and my colleagues while also providing a safe service. I'll admit I had huge anxiety at the start – not sleeping; wondering how I was going to home-school my children and continue my own job; worrying about what would happen to my husband's job as a dentist; worrying about my patients.

We had very little guidance from above until quite late, and by the time this came we had already made most of our own plans. I made some heartbreaking calls in those early months of the pandemic, to patients who had lost love ones and hadn't even been able to say goodbye. Some days I couldn't hold back the hot tears that persistently threatened to brim over. Sometimes it just felt so overwhelming, but, if there's one thing medics are good at, it is holding it together in a crisis (at least front of house – even if I did collapse in a heap when I got home).

As time went on, I became more at ease with telephone and video calls. However, there are some things we just cannot assess on the phone and in those cases, we needed to bring patients down to the surgery for a face-to-face review. We continued to do this all the way through the pandemic (despite the media reports suggesting otherwise). Systems were set up locally so that any patients with symptoms of Covid-19 were seen at 'hot sites' with vital signs being taken in car parks or special rooms that could be completely decontaminated, and special 'hot' visiting teams were deployed. Anyone else who needed to be assessed face-to-face we brought to the surgery within set timeframes to minimise the numbers of people in the waiting areas.

We started to (and continue to) wear PPE to see all patients. After a week of doffing and donning and cleaning the rooms after each patient, it soon seemed like second nature and just another part of the job. Seeing people face to face was really quite special. For some of them I was the first contact they had had in months. One mother told me that I was the only other person that had held her baby as I did the eight-week check – something that I would take for granted usually, but it suddenly seemed so precious. At times it was heartbreaking, telling someone they may have breast cancer and not being able to even reach out a hand or give them a hug if that was what they needed. I also found it hard to reconcile with the fact patients couldn't see my facial expressions. It made everything less human.

But we got through it. The team spirit was incredible. We laughed together, cried together and tried to find a way through. We learnt each other's strengths and supported each other's weaknesses like a family. The outpouring of support from our patients was also completely overwhelming – thanking us for being there, leaving hampers and chocolates. It was nice to feel appreciated, although sometimes it was bittersweet as I always wondered how long it would be before the tables turned and we would be scapegoated again.

In some ways work was a comfort – that familiarity and my last grasp of routine and normality in an otherwise upside-down world. A world where my children were being home-schooled and I was the teacher! Some days it was too much, too stifling, feeling that everyone was relying on me to have the answers and to keep things under control, when everything around me seemed to be spinning in the opposite direction.

I've learnt a lot and continue to do so. If someone had said to me, 'You will have to change your entire working practices overnight while home-schooling your kids while having no outside support,' I would have gone into a meltdown at the thought. But we did just that. I'm stronger than I thought I was. Now I feel like anything is possible and it's kind of exciting to embrace the changes in primary care – but gosh, I'm looking forward to the day I can hug my patients again!

14 July 2020
The government announces that wearing facemasks will become compulsory in shops and supermarkets from 24 July, following the lead of Scotland, who instituted these measures on 10 July [NHS PROVIDERS 2020].

17 July 2020
Captain Sir Tim Moore is knighted by the Queen at Windsor Castle [BBC 2020l].

20 July 2020
The University of Oxford's AstraZeneca vaccine is shown to trigger an immune

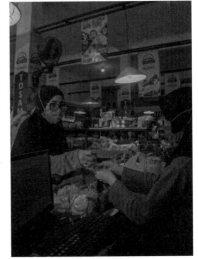

(Photo by Fiqri Aziz Octavian on Unsplash)

response in early trials. The UK has already ordered a million doses of the vaccine along with 90 million doses of the vaccines being developed by BioNTech and Pfizer [NHS Providers 2020].

29 July 2020
The Public Accounts committee criticises the government's decision to allow around 25,000 hospital patients in England to be discharged to care homes without Covid-19 tests at the start of the pandemic to free up hospital beds. Public Health England said that testing capacity was limited at the start of the crisis to only 3,500 tests per day and had to be prioritised for those in intensive care. Regular testing for staff and residents in care homes started earlier this month [PARLIAMENT PUBLICATIONS 2020].

30 July 2020
People testing positive for coronavirus are required to isolate for 10 instead of 7 days [PHE 2020b].

Hospital Security
Matthew Connop is an NHS Security Officer who works at the University Hospitals Birmingham Trust.

"The definition of a Security Officer is someone who is 'hired to patrol, guard and protect business, property and people from theft, vandalism and acts of abuse or violence'. Who would think that you would need security in a hospital? Someone to unlock doors perhaps, or someone to navigate a visitor's journey? But security… really? Why would we be needed in a hospital?

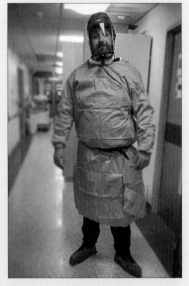

Matthew in PPE at work.

The Emergency Department is where we spend the majority of our time. 'Drunken louts who can't handle their alcohol' I hear you mutter. You would be so wrong in thinking that, let me assure you. We interact with different people every single shift. No two days are the same. From dealing with intoxication through drink and drugs, to mental health issues and attempted suicides. From highly delirious elderly people who have become aggressive due to an infection, to patients bought in by police for their own safety.

I have been assaulted, spat at, punched, kicked, bitten. I've gone home with black eyes and split lips. On one occasion I was threatened with a golf club and nearly ran over with a car – deliberately, all for doing my job. Verbal abuse is bad enough, but no one should be physically assaulted simply for trying to do their job and help people.

My medical colleagues also continue to be assaulted on a daily basis, as they do their jobs. They are sworn at, shouted at and, on occasions, physically assaulted – all for trying to make people better. Unless you work in a hospital setting, you would never believe what goes on.

We also have to attend other wards and departments to assist staff in administering medications such as sedation or simply to escort vulnerable people around the hospital site. Then there is the legal side to our position where, for a number of reasons, a patient may not legally leave or discharge themselves, we may face a sometimes physical struggle to stop them leaving. Next, comes the security part of our job. Locking and unlocking parts of the hospital, attending and dealing with fire alarm activation – great fun when you have to climb eight flights of stairs to the top of the block onto a ward where a patient has been smoking in the toilet and activated the sprinkler alarm system.

Some twelve-hour shifts are finished without a break, with hardly anything to drink and sometimes nothing to eat at all. Our pager likes to bleep to alert us to a situation occurring the second our food has pinged finished in the microwave – then its vest on and rush out the door, again.

The last four months have been horrendous for the NHS. Myself and my security colleagues assisted medical staff in transferring intubated patients up to ITU who didn't know whether they would ever wake up again. Returning the next night to find out many of these patients hadn't made it through the night will stay with me for a very long time. Due to the visiting restrictions put in place by Trust executives following government guidance, we were responsible for denying access to the relatives of dying and deceased patients. Denying them their last goodbye, their final kiss will haunt me forever.

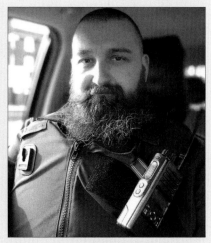

Matthew in his security vest.

I would never have dreamed that I would need to dress the way I did during the pandemic to be a hospital security officer. Full PPE, respiratory hood, masks, gloves, aprons, plastic shoe socks, arm and leg covers.

I also routinely wear a stab vest as the risk assessment deems it an essential piece of kit to try and keep me safe when on duty doing my job.

So, the pay is not the greatest and I am routinely assaulted, both verbally and physically, so why do I do it? I love my job and work with some amazing people every day. We have fun, we have laughs, we have tears and we have sadness, but if I can try to keep my colleagues safe while they are trying and help and care for everyone else, then I will continue to do so for as long as I can."

August

- 17,396,943 cases globally; 675,060 deaths
- 305,500 cases in the UK; 41,374 deaths
  (WHO 2020a, GOV.UK 2021)

Figure 1. Number of confirmed* COVID-19 cases reported in the last seven days by country, territory or area, 26 July to 1 August **

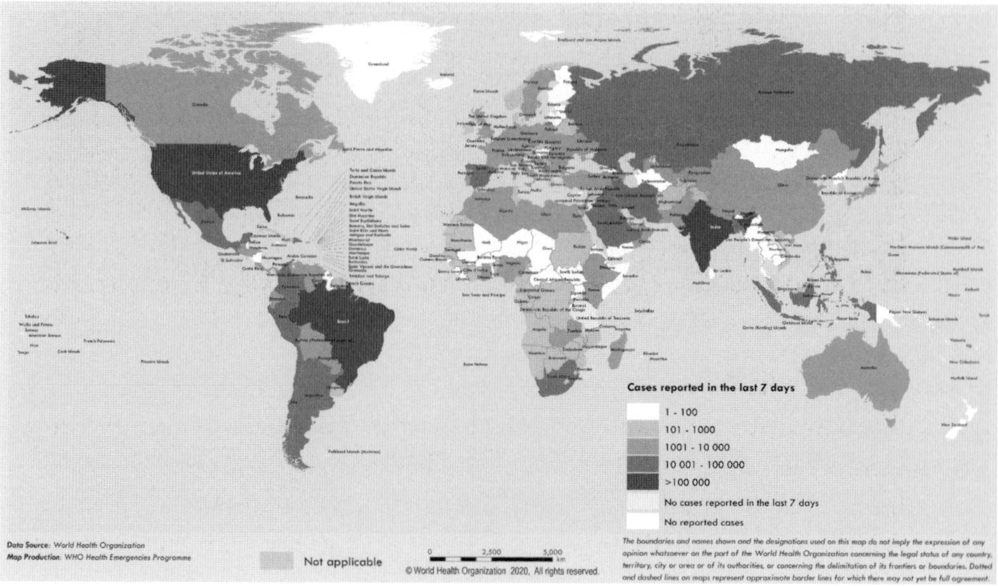

3 August 2020

The 'Eat Out To Help Out' scheme launches, in which restaurants and pubs offer half-price meals to customers during August, with the remainder of the cost picked up by the government [HM Revenue and Customs 2020].

5 August 2020

The Home Affairs committee admits that lack of border measures in the UK early in the pandemic was a mistake, and that the spread of Covid-19 could have been slowed by implementing quarantine measures. In February and early March, all passengers from Hubei Province in China and certain areas of South Korea, Iran and Italy were asked to self-isolate for 14 days on arrival into Britain. On 13 March an 'inexplicable' decision was made to end self-isolation for all international arrivals and limited only to those displaying any symptoms. It is likely that thousands of infected people arrived into the UK before lockdown started 10 days later [BBC 2020m].

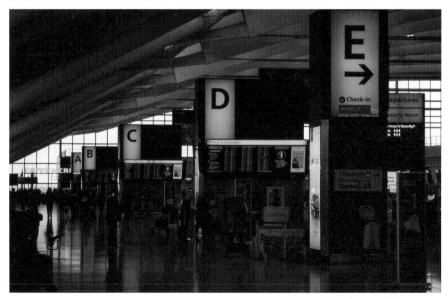

Heathrow Airport. (*Nick Fewings on Unsplash*)

12 August 2020
The Covid-19 death toll is reduced by over 5,000 due to a change in methodology. Previously, anyone who had tested positive for the virus before death was included in the figure, the new approach only records death due to Covid-19 if the person has a positive test within the last 28 days [PULSE 2020].

14 August 2020
Fines for refusing to wear a face mask increase to £3,200 [BFGP 2020].

17 August 2020
The government plans to replace Public Health England with a specialist pandemic unit due to dissatisfaction with performance during the pandemic [BFPG 2020]. The National Institute for Health Protection (NIHP) will start work immediately, but not be formalised until spring 2021, bringing together PHE, NHS Test and Trace and the Joint Biosecurity Centre (JBC) [DHSC 2020c]. The organisation will manage the UK's response to Covid-19 and wider public health threats. The numerous other roles of PHE, namely preventing ill health and reducing health inequalities will be 'absorbed into the wider NHS' [ROBERTS, M 2020].

Mental Health Care for Older Adults during the Pandemic

Emma Tyrrell is a Band 5 Staff Nurse working in a community hospital in NHS Forth Valley. She works on a ward which provides mental health care for older adults with dementia. This is her account of life at work during the pandemic.

"I have spent most of my nineteen-year nursing career caring for patients with dementia, a condition which can present many challenges – not only for the patient but also to those who provide their care.

When Covid-19 first hit the news, I have to admit that I really didn't pay it much more than passing attention. It was terrible of course, but it was all happening so far away. As the weeks progressed and the seasons turned, it became increasingly evident that this *was* going to affect us. In our spare moments at work, my colleagues and I would find ourselves gravitating towards the ward sitting room where the television would be on and we might catch an update on infection rates and deaths. We shook our heads in silent sympathy when we watched reports about the devastating situation in Italy … and then Spain … and we debated among ourselves how we thought we might keep ourselves, our families and our patients safe. It didn't matter what we talked about, the conversation would inevitably return to coronavirus. We felt anxious and frightened. We felt stressed. We would resume work after days off with an unsettling feeling of not knowing what situation we would be returning to.

NHS Forth Valley were sending out Covid-19 bulletins and updates on a frequent, almost daily, basis at first and the changes seemed to be coming so quickly that, sometimes, I wouldn't even read them as I fully expected the situation to very quickly change again. Guidelines for reporting Covid-related deaths, guidelines for non-Covid-related deaths, videos about how to carry out testing, videos on how to don and doff PPE, what PPE to use and when – it felt never-ending and, at times, I wished I could close my eyes and it would go away. At other times I felt a fierce sense of duty and pride for myself and my colleagues. We *would* do this, we *would* keep our patients safe and we would show everyone what stern stuff the NHS is made of. A rollercoaster of emotions and, thankfully, the latter has endured!

Our usual remit for the ward is to admit patients with a moderate to severe level of dementia who have already undergone a period of assessment and who require a further period of in-patient care before they might be ready to go to a nursing home or other long-term care arrangement. Our remit during peak pandemic was to admit patients with a milder level of dementia, and perhaps with more physical or medical needs than we were used to, in order to free up beds in Forth Valley Royal Hospital to allow them greater capacity to care for the expected influx of Covid-19 patients. We would not be admitting patients for treatment of Covid-19, but we would be instrumental in relieving the pressure on those who were.

A flurry of activity seemed to follow over the succeeding days and weeks, speeding up discharges for those who were ready and admitting those who weren't. Patients being admitted to us had already been tested as they had usually been in hospital for some time prior to transfer. Nursing homes were requesting, prior to accepting transfers from the ward, that patients be tested twice for Covid-19 and return two negative swabs. Due to their level of cognitive impairment our patients were often unable to give informed consent for the testing procedure. If the patient had an 'Adults With Incapacity' (AWI) form in place then we were able to carry out testing without their consent, but doing so might prove very challenging – how would we swab the throat of a patient who was repeatedly resisting us and refusing to open their mouth? It seemed more likely that the patient would not be tested and therefore remain with us. Fortunately, we were not presented with this situation and were able to perform the required tests by explaining the procedure in as simple terms as possible and by having extra staff on hand to soothe and reassure the patient if needed.

It soon became policy that we wear masks throughout our shift. This was the only right course of action but this was also a difficult transition for us. The therapeutic relationship between mental health nurse and patient relies heavily on non-verbal communication and the ability to appear non-threatening towards patients with severe cognitive impairment who may be confused, disorientated and frightened, and a smile goes a long way towards helping build this relationship. How would our patients react to not seeing our smiles and other facial expressions? How would they react to being approached by a masked figure in the semi-darkness of their bedroom at night as the nurses carried out their checks? Would the incidence of aggression rise? Would we see an increase in the levels of stress and distress in our patients? Our relationship with our patients felt especially important now as all but essential visiting had stopped when the country went into lockdown and our patients would not be seeing their family and friends for some time. We began to smile more, making sure this was reflected in the visible parts of our faces. We softened the tone of our voices and opened our postures. We used touch more, a reassuring hand on a patient's arm or shoulder, and we endeavoured to bring more into our conversations with them. Occasionally a patient might pass comment on our masks but it seemed that our efforts paid off and there did not appear to be an increase in any of the behaviours about which we had been concerned.

Another concern was how we would contain the virus if there was an outbreak on the ward. A notable feature of all the dementia wards in which I have worked is the number of patients who wander around the ward. They might be looking for something, perhaps seeking an exit, or their condition may cause the kind of restlessness which only the ability to be continually active can alleviate. Providing the patient isn't distressed this wouldn't normally be a concern, but allowing them to wander unhindered would be inappropriate in the event of an outbreak. Our patients generally have little concept of infection prevention and control procedures and social distancing is unfeasible in dementia wards for a variety of reasons, but how could we enforce isolation on a patient who was infected but who felt too well to be nursed in bed and who would not understand why their movements must be restricted? Could we reasonably isolate infected patients within their rooms and expect our therapeutic relationship to be unaffected and their sense of mental wellbeing to be maintained?

We asked these questions as mental health nurses, putting the mental health and wellbeing of our disorientated and vulnerable patients to the forefront – this perspective is in our nature. We are in the fortunate and most-likely uncommon position of not having identified (to date) a single case of Covid-19 in the ward, but we remain on our guard. We have begun to gravitate back to the sitting room and the television again to await news reports of 'the second wave' but we are okay, we are increasingly aware of our strengths and weaknesses and of those in our work environment and we are quietly preparing ourselves for what the coming months may present.

This is my own personal account. I am not presuming to speak for my colleagues, but I have used the word 'we' in many cases here because our team effort has endured, and we have supported each other throughout."

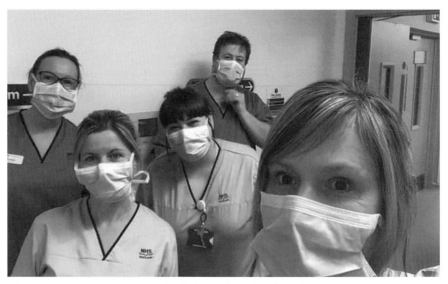

Mental Health nurses smiling behind the masks – first day of mask wearing.

Public Health in the UK

Our systems for communicable disease control have been slowly eroded and fragmented since the 1970s, when the role of Medical Officer for Health (MOH) was abolished. Historically, each locality employed a MOH, charged with public health responsibilities and access to local public health laboratories. This steering role was replaced by community physicians and then centralised, and the laboratories transferred to NHS hospitals.

In 2012, Public Health England was created to protect the public from disease, and local authorities were instructed to run it, serving 343 local authority areas in England from only nine regional hubs. It is no wonder contact tracing and testing was halted so early in the pandemic – the UK did not have the resources, expertise or manpower to do this.

Moving forwards, instead of being bound by generic centralised policies, our public health services need to be rebuilt with more involvement from experienced clinicians and more control for local teams to tailor their plans to their own communities.

The BAME GP

Dr Sonali Dutta-Knight is an Associate GP in Newcastle-Upon-Tyne. She founded the group Healthcare Professionals Against Racism and blogs as The BAME GP (https://medium.com/@thebamegp). The health disparities highlighted by the pandemic inspired this piece.

"The NHS is the UK's largest and arguably most diverse employer. The March 2019 Workforce report highlighted that 44 per cent of doctors and 21 per cent of nurses and other Allied Healthcare Staff are from Black, Asian and Minority Ethnic (BAME) backgrounds [NHS DIGITAL 2019]. Among the healthcare workers who have died from Covid-19, an analysis of media reports showed that 95 per cent of the doctors, 64 per cent of nurses and 63 per cent of Allied Healthcare Staff were from BAME backgrounds [COOK, T et al 2020].

Among the general population, the Office for National Statistics published data showing that being Black, Asian or Ethnic Minority in the UK is a serious risk factor for death due to Covid-19 disease, with a more than seven-fold increase in Black compared to White ethnicities [ONS 2020].

The prominence of such significant ethnic disparities has created unprecedented focus on racism in healthcare.

British Medical Training: 'The Best in the World'

Historically, there was a need for indigenous doctors in the Commonwealth countries and colonies, largely because there were not enough British doctors and it was decided that treatment of those 'lesser' races were best kept within their own.

The knowledge, culture and heritage of any countries belonging to the Empire were considered inferior, and medical training was not exempt from this. The indigenous training for doctors and healers that had pre-existed in the Empire was abolished and replaced by medical schools based on British styles. In the early nineteenth century in India, non-British doctors who lived there under British rule were only allowed to practice medicine formally if they collaborated by registering with the General Medical Council and sat exams based in London [ESMAIL, A. 2007].

The powerful propaganda that British medical training is superior persists to this day. Doctors who had trained and worked in Britain were held in high esteem in their countries of origin. Even pre-dating the NHS, there are historical records of BAME doctors and nurses working in the UK.

Many Jewish families escaping persecution in Europe in the early part of the twentieth century also fled to Britain and Jews first started to enter British medical schools during the First World War [COOPER, J. 2018]. Their experience of anti-Semitism was similar to the racism experienced by black and brown doctors and it is reported that many ended up in general practice and sometimes even anglicised their names to be able to find jobs. During the current pandemic, Jews have also been noted to have an increased risk of death from Covid-19 [ONS 2020].

The NHS and its workforce
The founding of the NHS in 1948 created demand for doctors, nurses and support staff. Recruitment drives in the Commonwealth and Colonies led to an influx of immigration and the first ship from the Caribbean, *The Empire Windrush*, arrived in Tilbury Docks on 22 June 1948. By the 1950s an estimated 3,000 overseas qualified doctors were working in the NHS [ESMAIL, A. 2007]. Throughout the 1960s and 70s, discrimination of ethnic minority doctors was commonplace and the antipathy from within the medical profession is displayed in the correspondence columns of the British Medical Journal. Almost every issue included letters from doctors complaining about language problems and the standard of education. The adverts page would commonly state that 'only British graduates need apply for vacant posts'. This practice was only stopped in 1976 when it was

deemed illegal following the introduction of the Race Relations Act [ESMAIL, A. 2007].

Many doctors and nurses who immigrated to the UK with specific career ambitions discovered they were unable to achieve their goals due to this systemic racism. Some returned to their home countries, but others stayed and continued working within the NHS. Many of those doctors aspired to work in secondary care as consultant physicians and surgeons but market forces dictated that those jobs went to white doctors first and many doctors ended up working in areas unwanted by their white colleagues.

Unfortunately, ethnic disparities persist to this day. The bar for racism has for too long been set as the violent actions of white supremacists, when in fact, unless we begin to address our own disconnection with history, we ignore our own unconscious complicity in health care inequalities and the persistence of both structural and unconscious bias. Unshakable false beliefs that there are racial differences in physiology continue to mask the brutal effects of discrimination and structural inequities, placing blame instead on individuals and their communities for statistically poor health outcomes.

Continued ethnic disparities in medical training were outlined in a 2020 BMJ review, which reported that doctors and medical students from ethnic minority backgrounds are up to three times as likely as their white counterparts to fail an examination [LINTON, S 2020]. In 2017 the pass rate in postgraduate examinations was 75 per cent among white students and 63 per cent among UK ethnic minority students. Among international medical graduates, the pass rate was 46 per cent for white students and 42 per cent for students from other ethnic groups [LINTON, S 2020]. In 2016 UK doctors from an ethnic minority background applying for consultant posts were both less likely to be shortlisted than white doctors (66 per cent versus 80 per cent) and less likely to be offered a post than white doctors (57 per cent versus 77 per cent); furthermore, basic pay for consultants from ethnic minority backgrounds was 4.9 per cent less than for white consultants in 2017 [LINTON, S 2020].

Ethnic minority doctors are twice as likely to be referred to the GMC. For doctors who trained outside the UK, that figure increases

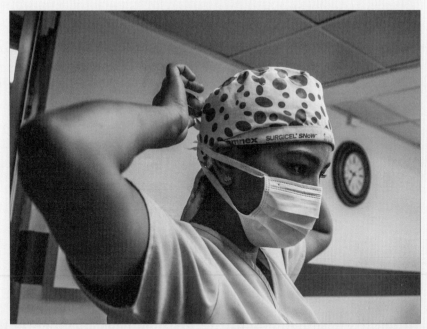

(Photo by SJ Objio on Unsplash)

to two-and-a-half times more likely [MAJID, A. 2020]. Analysis by the GMC of why this occurs highlights a pervasive 'outsider' dynamic in the NHS. They report that 'doctors perceived as lower status outsiders – such as doctors trained outside the UK – are not given the support they need by bosses and colleagues and are more likely to end up being blamed and facing disciplinary action when things go wrong.'

The report goes on to say that ethnic minority doctors 'are also over-represented in roles that can isolate them, such as in locum posts or in small or demanding general practices, leaving them more vulnerable to complaints' [GMC 2019]. A culture of fear also means that ethnic minority doctors are more likely to be bullied [NHS England 2019] and feel less confident about raising concerns for fear of a backlash. During the Covid-19 pandemic, the BMA reported that BAME doctors were less likely to have access to adequate PPE compared to their white counterparts [COOPER, K. 2020]. Similar findings were found for BAME nurses [ROYAL COLLEGE OF NURSING 2020]."

Ethnic disparities for patients

Many ethnic disparities in health outcomes have for years, been attributed to scientifically debunked racial 'physiological differences'. There are, however, areas that cannot be explained by these reasons at all. For example, black women are five times more likely to die and Asian women are almost twice as likely to die than white women in the first six weeks after having a baby according to the 2014-16 Confidential Inquiry into Maternal Deaths report [KNIGHT M et al 2018]. The women involved have spoken about their experiences, with a common theme being they were not listened to, and symptoms were downplayed [KASPRZAK, E. 2019]. The BMJ reported in 2020, that ethnic minority patients receive worse mental healthcare than white patients, which the Race Equality Foundation attributed to ethnic bias [THORNTON J. 2020]; while a 2013 review of racial disparities in pain management found that pain and its treatment are strongly influenced by race and ethnicity [WYATT, R. 2013].

Medical training textbooks and websites to this day continue to primarily feature images of illness in white skin. Many of these texts remain highly respected and are exported around the world. This is thought to be the reason that doctors find it harder to diagnose conditions in patients with darker skin tones [MCFARLING, U.L. 2020]. This knowledge gap may have contributed to increased BAME deaths due to Covid-19 due to the paucity of images of the skin manifestations of the disease in darker skin [LESTER JC, et al 2020]. People with darker skin tones simply do not look 'blue' when their oxygen levels are low, meaning that healthcare staff miss a vital clinical clue. It has even been suggested that peripheral oxygen saturation monitors may encode racial bias as they were developed on white populations and give less accurate readings in people of colour when they have low oxygen levels [MORAN-THOMAS, A. 2020].

Covid-19 and the Black Lives Matters marches have highlighted the need to review racial disparities and examine our own complicity in structural racism and unconscious bias. It is clear there is a long record of racism in British History and within the NHS. We must begin to look at ways that we can truly reduce these disparities, for our colleagues and patients alike.

September

- 26,121,999 cases globally; 864,618 deaths
- 337,168 cases in the UK; 41,655 deaths

(WHO 2020a, GOV.UK 2021)

1 September 2020
The majority of schools in England, Wales and Northern Ireland reopen. UK Chief Medical Officers reaffirmed in August that children are at low risk of contracting and dying from Covid-19 [BFPG 2020].

9 September 2020
Facebook states it will not remove anti-vaccine posts, despite concerns over echo chambers of misinformation [BFPG 2020]. (In Feb 2021 Facebook does go on to ban posts containing false claims about vaccines [PAUL, K 2021].

Covid affected the entire planet. What follows are personal accounts from healthcare workers around the globe, which help put our experience in the NHS into context.

A Siege Within a Siege: Covid-19 in Gaza
Dr Natalie Thurtle is an Emergency Physician, formerly NHS, now based in Sydney. She is currently the Medical Coordinator for Médecins Sans Frontières (Doctors Without Borders) in Palestine. She explores some of the challenges of responding to Covid-19 in a low resource setting with a population already living under severe restrictions.

"In March 2020, a meme was circulating…
    'Dear World, how is the lockdown? Love Gaza.'
    On 11 March 2020, Covid-19 was labelled a pandemic and the global adrenaline surge translated into many countries halting daily life and implementing 'lockdowns'. This approach was mostly tolerated at first, as action was required in the face of an ill-defined biological threat. As the disease undulated across the globe and stretched out into a second year, accompanied by an 'infodemic' [THE LANCET ID 2020] and by highly politicised rhetoric, the use of lockdowns has

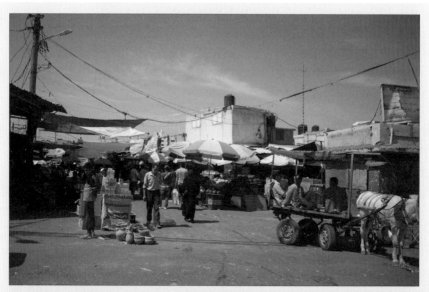

Daily life in a small market in Gaza. (*Copyright Aurelie Baumel/MSF May 2018*)

become more controversial. The discourse is flamed by lack of data on how to optimise the use of lockdowns to mitigate health-care system overwhelm, and on the magnitude of their unintended consequences in specific settings.

The loudest voices on this topic are often from socio-economic strata where the collateral impacts of lockdown are potentially more easily withstood, conflating public health measures with an attack on freedom. In Gaza, and in other contexts with fragile economies and infrastructure, the threat from Covid-19 versus the consequences of lockdown presents an impossible line to walk.

Gaza has a population of 2 million living in a strip 45km long and at its maximum 10km wide. Residents have lived under siege since 2007, meaning that borders, airspace and waters as well as imports and exports are tightly controlled by Israel. There are frequent airstrikes and escalations in conflict with Israel. There is resultant severe poverty and well documented socioeconomic decay in Gaza, with over 50 per cent of the population living below the poverty line and an unemployment rate of approximately 50 per cent [UNCTAD 2020].

In the context of Covid-19, the siege proved initially beneficial. A lack of porous borders kept the in-flow of the virus controlled, in conjunction with swift and stringent action from the authorities. Entrants to Gaza underwent institutional quarantine for 21 days. There was no community transmission reported in March or April, or even in July. Could Gaza achieve the holy grail of total suppression until community vaccination roll-out?

No.

Community transmission was first identified at the end of August 2020 and by November, Gaza was diagnosing over a thousand cases per day on PCR, with an almost 50 per cent positivity rate due to their limited testing capacity. Months of preparations from the Ministry of Health and international agencies lurched to life, but the tissue paper health infrastructure afforded by the longstanding siege quickly groaned. On 22 November 2020 WHO declared 'within one week we will not be able to care for critical cases' [AL-MUGHARABI, N 2020].

Médecins Sans Frontières (MSF) worked alongside the Ministry of Health (MoH) supporting the MoH team by providing senior critical care clinicians; training junior staff; developing patient flow protocols and donating drugs and consumables. Many other agencies also provided support and donated items including equipment for both non-invasive and mechanical ventilation and large-scale oxygen concentrators. Projection of need through modelling was extraordinarily challenging, as it has been worldwide. When will the wave come, how big will it be, how long will it last, what will the critical care and mortality burden be? These questions which pose a challenge even for high-resource contexts, could not be deduced meaningfully for Gaza.

Gaza MoH is de facto donation-dependent, and hence reliant on what individual entities and the Health Cluster feel willing and able to donate. Oxygen sources are limited, with incendiary risk a key concern during 'normal' times due to regular escalations in conflict. Relevant supply chains were disrupted, price gouged and flowing with fakery, and complicated by the Israeli occupation. This donation-dependent paradigm shines a light not only on the occupation, but on the impact

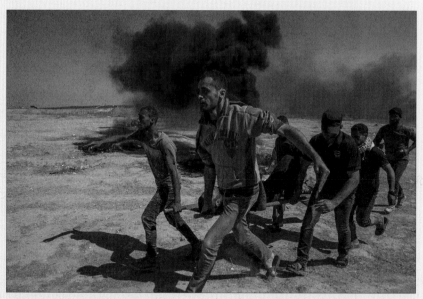

Demonstration in Gaza – evacuating the wounded. (*Copyright Laurence Geal/MSF. May 2018*)

of humanitarian response in Gaza. This so-called Humanitarian Paradox, whereby long-term patchwork emergency offerings, while meant well, may contribute to the lack of infrastructure and strategic planning [HAMMOUDEH, W 2020].

Misinformation and disinformation regarding Covid-19 in the era of the 'Infodemic' is no less prevalent in Gaza than elsewhere, with ubiquitous access to social media platforms and a deep mistrust of public messaging from years of political tension. Even among health staff there were initial cries of a hoax. Some feared that Covid-19 was an excuse to contain the population during angst related to Israel's ongoing annexation of the West Bank and other perceived political failures by the authorities. In early December, residents of Hebron, one of the worst hit areas in the West Bank, held anti-lockdown protests against the Palestinian Authority, similar to those witnessed all over the world.

In Gaza, enthusiasm for lockdown was even lower, given the decades long siege and the well-documented impact of existing curtailments – not just on daily life but also on access to medical care, education and other human rights. The de facto authority Hamas resisted initiating lockdown even at the end of November, finally capitulating as The

United Nations (UNRWA) flagged imminent health system collapse amid a rupture of PCR tests in early December.

Between the first identified community transmission in August, until December 2020, Gaza tried to manage with a local lockdown model (after a brief generalised lockdown), barricading areas where clusters of cases were identified. The population density and nature of transmission meant it couldn't hold. As testing collapsed and cries of imminent overwhelm sounded from UN bodies and the Gaza Coronavirus Taskforce, Gaza reactively slammed into brief, snap lockdowns with the hope of averting collapse of the healthcare system, nothing more would be tolerated. There was concern that it was too little, too late.

As of 4 February 2021, Gaza has a 1.0 per cent case fatality rate for Covid-19. 527 of 52,048 cases have died.

Data of total monthly deaths and excess death analysis is not publicly available for Gaza. This means that there are likely to be unidentified Covid-19 deaths, in the context of stretched testing capacity and frightened or misinformed patients not presenting for medical care and dying at home. Anecdotes also suggest a cohort of patients with means who are committed to managing their disease at home, organising home CPAP/BiPAP (breathing support) and oxygen. It is highly unlikely, however, that there is unnoticed mass mortality in Gaza related to Covid-19.

Studies regarding the global infection fatality rate (IFR) for the virus seem to be gathering around a figure of 0.5-1 per cent [VAN ASTEN, L ET AL 2021, WHO 2020d]. Gaza, with its young population, may have an IFR <1%, assuming the health service remains functional.

With 50 per cent of the population at or below the poverty line, the loss of even one day's earnings can have a detrimental impact on a family's health. The deterioration of the micro-economy from hard lockdowns stings the population.

Those in the humanitarian aid sector are, or should be, sensitised to the impact of colonialism on the paradigm in which we try to address health inequities. Covid-19 has exposed this in a multitude of ways, but not least the expectation that all must be dropped for or usurped by Covid-19 because of an IFR of 1 per cent.

A 0.5-1 per cent mortality over time, mostly impacting the elderly, may, unfortunately be tolerable in some contexts on a balance of risks assuming an inevitably slow vaccine roll-out, as opposed to aggressive or long lockdowns. Unfortunately, the data generally do not exist to support country-specific courses of action in low- to middle-income countries, so authorities are flying blind, including in Gaza, balancing impossible risks, as well as being at the mercy of the temptations of politicisation.

Preliminary findings from a seroprevalence study in January 2021, including a sample of 6,000 Palestinians suggests a seroprevalence of 40 per cent, however the full report is pending [UNITED NATIONS 2021].

Covid-19 is a fresh wound in the flesh of the health of the population of Gaza, but it must not be all consuming. Globally, it's key that the restrictions are not worse than the disease. Humanitarian agencies must be careful not to apply a Western lens to the issue, or to support a representation of the risks which is not locally tailored."

Gaza, February 2021.

The South African Experience – Covid-19 in the Private Sector

Dr Arina de Bruin is a doctor with a special interest in aviation, maritime and telemedicine, currently working in the private sector of the South African healthcare system.

"I had never imagined that my world would come crashing down. The fact that it was the ACTUAL world that seemed to erupt into chaos was really a bit of a relief – at least I wasn't being melodramatic.

It's easy to imagine that a doctor should be used to death; I mean, we see it all the time, right? It's not new, it's not personally damaging, and it most certainly shouldn't impact how we practice. It's our job for goodness sake. In theory, this is all true, except for the fact that life does matter, every single life that you save, but most certainly every life that you don't.

I am 29 years old, a relative spring chicken in the world of medicine, but living through a pandemic makes you re-evaluate your stance on what is construed as your physical age, and how old you are based on your actual life experience. I emphatically remember sitting in our office during a sixteen-hour night shift and watching as Covid-19 was declared a pandemic. I recall thinking to myself, 'They really are overreacting a bit now.' That was my age, and not my experience speaking.

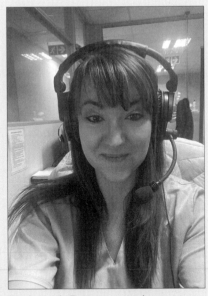

Dr Arina de Bruin wearing her telemedicine headset.

I graduated from medical school at the University of Pretoria in 2015 and was thrown into what I believed was the deep end for my two years of internship and one year of community service. After that I spent just under a year working in the intensive care unit of Chris Hani Baragwanath Academic Hospital in Johannesburg, (the biggest hospital in Africa and fourth largest in the world) and obtained my Diploma in Anaesthetics in the same year. Looking back, I realise that it was a mentally and emotionally taxing time, chipping away at my compassion and sense of humanity. While in the thick of it, I was mostly determined to do the best that I could with the often scanty resources available to me. By the end of the year I had to leave the unit to preserve what little sanity I had left. I did some serious introspection to make peace with the fact that I can't save everyone.

Doctors aren't superhuman – we are just trained to deal with challenging circumstances, and are exposed to these circumstances more often than everyone else. A professor in medical school once told me that the only difference between me and Joe Soap when coming across a motor vehicle accident by the side of the road, is that I'm used to seeing that amount of blood.

I had high hopes for 2020. I had just started a new relationship, and we were planning on traveling to Croatia in May for a holiday. My new job, where I telephonically talked flight crew through in-flight emergencies via Sat Com, was stimulating and interesting, and I was on my way to becoming flight ready. This meant that I would be transporting critically ill patients, putting my hard-won skills from ICU to good use. My expectation for the year changed when the story broke about a SARS-like virus that had originated from a small city in China, a place I had never even heard of.

Wuhan-City and its animal markets are now infamous, but I needed to pull up a Google map to find it at first. Every day the infection rate climbed, and every day I felt like the world was reacting to the reaction of itself. Surely, if the US is implementing this plan then the UK must do the same, especially seeing as Korea has done something similar and Japan was already thinking up a new strategy. Once again, my innocence surfaced. I was convinced that SARS-CoV-2 was gaining clout based purely on the fact that we now had access to social media to report the disastrous spread. Part of me still believes that social media played a role in the drama that surrounded the initial outbreak, and that it was sensationalised to an extent. You didn't need to be a reputable reporter to report on Covid-19.

South Africa (my home and my patriotic pride) remained serenely untouched by the devastation. My job, which is mostly internationally based, however, became increasingly difficult. We began fielding calls from airlines asking about patients on board the flight that had coughed two to three times, or had developed a borderline fever. Was this early Covid-19? Our advice protocols changed almost daily, and the South African Government began to ready itself for the worst-case scenario. The unfortunate truth is that in a population that deals with a large percentage of immune suppression, a rampant virus with no cure and very little resources for intervention could spell the ultimate catastrophe.

The reality only hit home for me when my boyfriend (who is a travelling cameraman) got sent back to South Africa from his international shoot, because the television series that he was filming was being postponed due to Covid-19. Selfishly, I was ecstatic to have my boyfriend home early, even if it meant that he was losing income. I walked into our home on his first night back with a fluttering heart, but was sorry to see that he looked a bit under the weather.

He had been travelling continuously for thirty-four hours through four different airports in three different countries, and appeared drained. I doctored him as best I could (it is what I do after all) and ascribed his lethargy to the commotion of international roaming. At this point, South Africa had just declared its first Covid-19 patient, a gentleman who had been skiing in Italy and returned with mild flu symptoms. He was pestered by media and healthcare workers alike, wanting to know what this new virus felt like. His treating physician was later diagnosed, and the spread was further tracked from there.

I continued on normally for the next few days, going to the office and working intermittent clinical shifts in various emergency departments, all the while hearing phenomenal stories about how the government was prepping for the possible explosive spread of Covid-19. The Chris Hani Baragwanath Hospital freed up an entire ward for possible Covid-19 patients; sourced fourteen ventilators and had their whole anaesthetic department providing rotating cover through these wards. All elective surgeries were cancelled, elective clinic dates postponed, and new screening protocols were implemented before admission to hospital in both the private and the public sectors.

I watched with interest as the country readied itself and assuaged the fears of my boyfriend who was still feeling unwell, later capitulating and referring him for a Covid-19 test as reassurance. His test came back unexpectedly positive. Suddenly the rose-coloured glasses turned an alarming shade of grey. What if I had wandered around and unwittingly caused some of my patients to fall ill? I felt irresponsible for not even considering Covid-19 as a diagnosis when he first returned. At the time, there was very little information available, and it had barely made the national news as anything other than a dark cloud on the horizon. It never crossed my mind that it might be living with us, under the same roof. Since his homecoming my boyfriend had only interacted closely with one friend and another family member – who both developed flu-like symptoms but both tested negative. I always remained completely asymptomatic, therefore never qualified for testing as per our protocols (to try and prevent a test kit shortage, a situation that had befallen many of our international friends). I am convinced that he was just shedding dead virus by the time that he arrived home and was no longer infectious.

Unfortunately the limitation of the test is that it can't determine whether the viral RNA that it is picking up is alive or not, so I can't be sure if I am correct, or if my guilty conscience is simply looking for a haven.

We were both immediately placed in self-isolation, but instead of feeling caged, this let me experience the pandemic from a whole new perspective. I was privy to the initial non-medical management of Covid-19 positive patients by our Department of Health and National Institute for Communicable Disease (NICD). We deduced that he was patient number 159, based on a list published by the NICD indicating the demographics of the positive patients. I was in absolute awe of the level of concern and professionalism that was executed by both governing authorities. He was phoned at least once every two days by an appointed person who was following up on his symptoms and 'chasing' all of his close contacts, to be able to monitor them in turn. They made sure that we had access to food and medicine, and continuously counselled us on which danger signs to look out for and when to seek advanced medical attention. I may have badgered him about his physical health more than was necessary, but from what I could tell and what he relayed, he had only mild symptoms. He never suffered from shortness of breath or a fever, and he only experienced a dry cough and malaise. It was reassuring to see that he recovered fully, and that he did so quickly.

It was on day nine of our fourteen-day self-isolation period that our president addressed the nation and told us that a three-week lockdown of the country was being instituted. He was inspiring, and the whole nation breathed a collective sigh of relief that we, a small third world country, were handling the situation on par with the rest of the world. As a health care worker, I thought that the lockdown would have very little effect on my life once my isolation period was over, since I was permitted to travel to work as usual. Abstract fears were mitigated when the population understood that everyone was still allowed to purchase essential items and even travel if it was deemed crucial. The streets were quieter, the queues in the grocery stores were shorter, and the foot traffic was less intimidating. Once again, my age let me slip into the comfortable illusion of a 'better' circumstance. My obliviousness to the severity of the impact the lockdown had on our country came crashing down when my own father had to take a 50 per cent decrease in his salary; and my freelance boyfriend was now not allowed outside of our house to generate an income.

The number of in-flight emergencies had decreased so drastically (because the number of flights was essentially non-existent) that our operational hours were cut by two thirds. The emergency rooms that I worked at part-time also cut their staffing down because no 'green codes' were attending these hospitals and generating revenue, which ultimately led to my own salary decreasing by 20 per cent. This was an absolutely foreign concept to me, a doctor in the private sector that had to take a pay cut because of low volumes of patients in the middle of a pandemic. In the public sector it seemed that the trend was holding, with empty wards and bored specialists. In an effort to 'flatten the curve' we had managed to flatten our economy as well.

After a couple of weeks, our numbers of Covid-19 positive cases began to increase drastically, necessitating the lockdown to be extended by another two weeks (a total of five weeks of what we now think of as 'hard lockdown'), and numbers peaked in three of our provinces. Even with the higher patient volume, the lockdown still prohibited any possibility of reviving the hospitality and entertainment industries.

Horror stories of doctors having to decide which patients to resuscitate, which patients to admit, and even of patients stealing each other's oxygen began to surface. That being said, my personal experience of treating suspected or known Covid-19 patients differed very little from what I was used to seeing in the units I worked at. We now had cordoned-off sections dedicated to high-risk persons under investigation (PUIs), and we had to don PPE for each of those patients, which took some extra time, but my patient profile remained mostly the same. The biggest impact was that even hospitals were now practicing social distancing, with many departments having a diminished bed capacity, ultimately meaning tha t the decreased number of patients we were able to admit rapidly led to overflows into the actual emergency departments. Despite this, all of my patients were kind and understanding of the situation.

I did have one terrible encounter where a patient was deemed a 'PUI' because he was suffering from shortness of breath. He was taken to the dedicated smaller area where I could go and see him once I was wearing all of my PPE. I quickly determined that he was short of breath because he was having a heart attack, and wanted

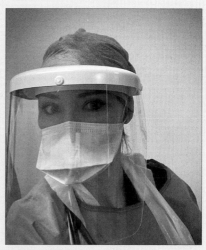

Dr Arina de Bruin in PPE.

to move him into our resuscitation area. Unfortunately, there was already a non-PUI patient in the area, and there was a second ventilated patient in the separate room next to him. This meant that my patient couldn't be moved to an area that was deemed 'clean' because he could potentially infect the other healthy patients, even if this was the best area for him to be in. While I was busy sorting through the red tape to get him transferred and initiating his treatment, he deteriorated and coded (went into cardiac arrest). We performed CPR on him for almost an hour, but ultimately had to make the decision to stop resuscitation. There was a clear flaw in the system, but one that I was not in a position to overcome. Just the recollection of that night still gives me a sharp pang in my chest, and makes my heart beat a little bit faster. Even if his death wasn't necessarily preventable, I wanted to be able to do more to help him.

With the influx in patient numbers, be it mild flu-like symptoms or dangerous acute respiratory distress syndrome, the Department of Health and NICD couldn't follow-up with patients the way they had with my boyfriend anymore. Information about the virus was much more readily available anyway, and emergency hotline numbers were now being used. In the public sector there was news of ICUs being closed, mainly due to decreased bed capacity. There was a big effort to separate out potential Covid-19 cases from those that clearly had no relation, but we couldn't take any chances with the number of asymptomatic cases that were being recorded. My experience was that the discrepancy in patient volumes from those affected by Covid-19 was not really socio-economically based, but rather regionally.

The provinces that were hit the hardest were affected equally in both private and public sectors, where other areas of the country held firm in the belief that the virus was only contractible by a certain demographic, or if you moved into a specific area. This way of thinking was partially helped (and hindered) by the fact that we were not allowed inter-provincial travel, so the outbreaks remained relatively contained. The dynamic shifted fairly quickly, and as far as I am aware we were not stretched beyond our resources for very long, and not much more so than one would expect over say the festive season due to motor vehicle accidents or community assaults, under normal circumstances.

The company that I work for was one of the few frontrunners that had already instituted a Telemedicine platform before Covid-19 was a household term. During the pandemic, they affiliated with a laboratory to provide Covid-19 testing, including a doctor's telephonic consult if you tested positive, to counsel you on what to expect, how to self-isolate and for how long, and reassure you of the statistics. I was very eager to get involved in this and read up extensively on Covid-19 to be able to give accurate and appropriate information to patients who were scared and confused by all the fake news circulating on social media.

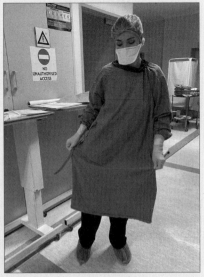

The volume of 'normal' patients started picking up as we had a phased release of lockdown, gradually allowing for alcohol, clothing and other industries to reopen. I was shocked when I realised what an impact alcohol sales specifically had had on our patient numbers in the emergency

Dr Arina de Bruin at work.

department. Sale of alcohol had been banned during lockdown and when it was reintroduced, I was working a clinical shift in an emergency department that is notorious for its gang violence. The amount of trauma cases we had in that one night was more than we had seen in the entire week before the restrictions lifted.

As the borders reopened and people started interacting with each other again, there was a definite increase in the number of active Covid-19 cases, despite ongoing restrictions.

Our mortality rate continued to hover around 2 per cent of infected cases, much lower than what was predicted. There were even a few studies trying to determine why we didn't seem to be as severely affected in terms of bad outcomes. There was speculation that the BCG vaccine played a role, but those hypotheses were later discounted. The country was starting to get restless, sensing economic collapse, with relief funds barely touching sides in terms of helping those in need. There was a lot of pressure put on governing bodies to lift restrictions and allow freedom of movement again, despite the risk of instigating a second wave of the pandemic. As it stands (in September 2020) we are still not allowed international travel, and we still have a curfew in place in the late evening to early morning.

Personally, I have both gained and lost from living through this pandemic. During hard lockdown and our self-isolation period I grew closer to my partner, and we built a solid foundation for what was at that point still a new relationship. I was able to ascertain how I deal with adversity and realise that I could cope with the pressures of medicine when there was very little that anyone else could do to help or support me. I realised that I am proud to do the work that I love. I also learned that there is a great misconception of the medical field and of doctors on the whole by the general public. When you feel like the world is collapsing, you realise that we are not machines that are unaffected by death, even if the patient was only known to us for a few minutes. Just because we see it more, doesn't make us immune to the finality of it. Yes, we chose to do this work, which can be extremely rewarding, but it can also be devastating. Nothing could have prepared us for the emotion associated with living through a pandemic, the sense of desolation or the waves utter joy that we experienced.

As a medical community, we all take pride in our work with our patients, but also in how we can communicate with their families and bring strength and hope to a community that can easily become forlorn. I grasped that nothing in life is a given, and that we have to celebrate the small victories with those around us, be it a loved one or a friendly stranger. Most of all, I discovered that the human race is still filled with humanity, with compassion and care and selflessness. We crave interaction, and we can be creative about how we obtain it. We are strong and resilient, and though we lose sight of our good intentions on occasion, we can, and from now on we will, do better. It seems that the world had to come crashing down to be extraordinarily rebuilt."

The South African Experience – In the Ganglands of the Cape Flats

Dr Randall Ortel is a family medicine registrar, and the first medical doctor to hail from the Manenberg community of Cape Town. He continued to work in his South African community throughout the pandemic and tells us about his experiences making a difference there.

Manenberg is a township on the Cape Flats region of Cape Town, South Africa. It was created in 1966 by the apartheid government for coloured* families as a result of a series of forced removals in which millions of non-white residents were taken from Cape Town central and dumped in townships built on the Cape Flats, with poor amenities and no transport links. Today, an estimated 56,301 residents live in the distinctive rows of red-roofed government three-storey housing blocks where conditions are often overcrowded, and the incidence of violent drug crime is high [WENGER, M. 2016].

The area is renowned for gang activity reporting a staggeringly high murder rate in 2018 of 108 per 100,000 [THOMAS, K et al 2018], making it among the most violent places in the world. More than ten large gangs and up to forty smaller ones are thought to operate in Manenberg, which covers an urban area of only 3.35 square kilometers. Education rates are low, with a reported 78 per cent of high school students dropping out, and unemployment is rife, with

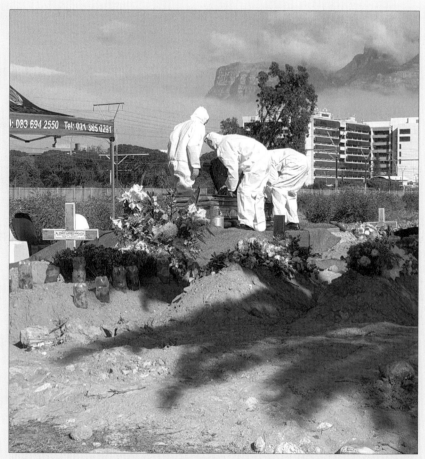

A Covid funeral takes place in the shadow of Table Mountain. (*Randall Ortel, with permission*)

only 64 per cent of working-age people employed [THOMAS, K et al 2018]. An unemployed, uneducated population of young people with time on their hands provides a willing recruitment pool for local gangs, which provide a source of both income and identity.

Dr Randall Ortel was born and bred in Manenberg and once dreamt of becoming a taxi driver or a garbage collector. After being awarded a bursary to study at Rhodes High School in neighbouring Mowbray his life changed direction. 'I always attained high marks before, but the standards were much higher at this school. It was here I decided to become a doctor, and I have never looked back.' Randall went on to study medicine at Stellenbosch University, and qualified as

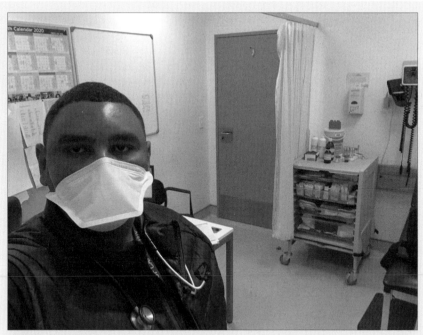

Dr Ortel in Clinic.

an emergency and occupational medicine practitioner. He is currently studying for his masters in family medicine.

'When you say you are from Manenberg, people look at you in a prejudiced way.' He says, 'their jaws drop. But Manenberg is the best springboard and it's a supportive community.' Randall continues to live in Manenberg, not because he has to but because he wants to, so he can provide a voice for his community.

Randall has become an important local figure, known affectionately as 'Doc' and understands the dynamics of the area. He regularly engages with the government and organisations implementing projects in Manenberg to advocate for his neighbours and local residents. When the Covid-19 crisis began to unfold, his community reached out to him, and Dr Ortel facilitated the care coordination of those testing positive for the virus.

'Manenberg is really densely populated' says Dr Ortel. 'It is common for twenty people to share one bathroom, which obviously does not help in terms of social distancing.' He found that many hospital colleagues failed to appreciate this when discharging Covid-19 positive patients back to Manenberg, that this group typically have no space to self-isolate. This prompted him to become actively involved in his local response to the outbreak. He spoke with community leaders so that when they heard of any positive cases, Randall could, with their permission, go and chat with them, check their results on the national laboratory system, and arrange appropriate quarantine. 'The community is so close knit that if someone gives me an address, I already know the circumstances in which they are living – and that opportunity is priceless.'

At the start of the pandemic, the community appeared defiant to government advice to outsiders, with poor uptake of mask wearing and sanitising. 'Sadly, with the ongoing shootings and gang violence, people feel they are at greater risk of being hit by a bullet than contracting Covid-19.' said Randall. He managed to work with local health services to disseminate public health information to the community in an understandable way. He set up WhatsApp groups where he hosted question and answer sessions with links to videos, and he carried out home visits to elderly residents and spoke to them about their concerns.

Randall also played a major role in calming some of the panic that arose from the pandemic. He describes how a ward councillor

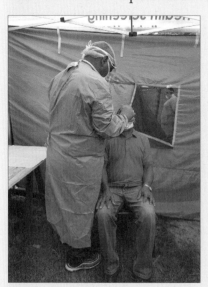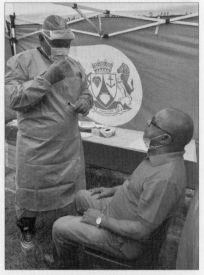

Dr Ortel swabbing a member of the community for Covid-19. (*Randall Ortel*)

contacted him for assistance dealing with a community protest. Residents had gathered outside the house of a woman with suspected Covid-19 and were victimising her, fearing she was roaming the streets and infecting their children. Randall accompanied this patient to a meeting with the councillor where it emerged she had been sent home from work due to another staff member testing positive. She had not been tested herself, but did have symptoms of fever and sore throat. She was taken to a local community hospital and diagnosed with an upper respiratory tract infection with suspected Covid-19, and discharged to isolate at home while awaiting her results.

The community members spotted her the next morning and again began to protest, alleging she had run away from hospital. Randall was asked to visit again to liaise and this time visited the patient at home. He found twenty-two people living on the property with the patient, with the patient herself sharing a 3x3m shack space with her two children and elderly mother, with no windows for ventilation. The patient agreed to be quarantined should she test positive and agreed to remain at home while awaiting results. Another two days later,

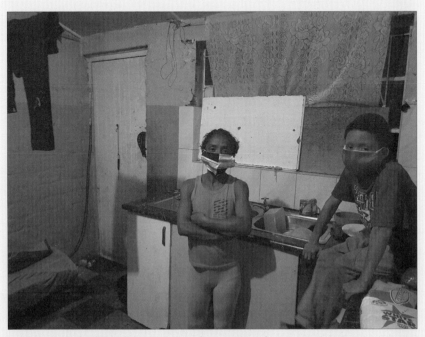

A Manenberg family isolating at home. (*Randall Ortel*)

the crowd complained again that the patient was roaming around. Randall again visited and found that the patient was struggling to handle the stigma at home and was trying to go to stay with her paternal grandmother (a high-risk patient herself). With consent, Randall checked her results, which she didn't yet have back, and found out she was Covid-19 positive. She was tearful, but agreed to be quarantined, which Randall was able to arrange for her.

The work Randall has done during the pandemic was entirely voluntary. 'It is a gang-ridden community, so it's not very safe,' he says. 'It's an absolute pleasure to serve my community, and to bring in much needed resources and skills. The beautiful part of it all is doing home visits, which have long been banned, and are especially needed for palliative care patients.'

* In South Africa, many mixed-race people prefer to use the term 'coloured' to describe themselves.

The Australian Experience

Dr Elaine Tennant is a British-trained doctor, specialising in Infectious Diseases and Public Health. She works in New South Wales, Australia, and divides her time between clinical and public health work.

"In late December 2019, an epidemiologist colleague forwarded an email from ProMED (a global surveillance system for infectious diseases), informing us that a novel coronavirus had been detected in Wuhan, China. I gave it a passing thought as I was distracted with work on a measles outbreak that we were managing at the time. Life was busy and we were all reeling from the terrible bushfire season that Australia was experiencing. Many rural communities had lost their homes. There had been huge loss of flora and fauna and our children had been restricted in outside play for several weeks due to the thick air pollution. These events had galvanised many of us to take more action on climate change during 2020 and I was hoping for a quieter year following a bit of upheaval during 2019. Little did we all know the carnage that would unfold.

I write this now in January 2021, and as things stand there have been over 90 million cases and nearly 2 million recorded deaths globally. I feel incredibly lucky to live in Australia at the moment, where we have recorded a total of around 28,000 cases and fewer than 1,000 deaths. This is still too many, but at this point the UK have recorded over 3 million cases and over 83,000 deaths [JOHN HOPKINS UNIVERSITY 2021]. My heart is aching for friends, family and colleagues who are currently there.

Australia and China have tight economic links and are geographically relatively close. Australia's Covid-19 experience could therefore very easily have been large in scale. Our first cases were detected fairly early in the course of the pandemic, in late January, just a few days before the WHO declared the outbreak a 'public health emergency of international concern'. These initial Covid-19 infected patients were isolated quickly. On 1 February, the Australian government closed the border to all travellers from mainland China, apart from Australian citizens/permanent residents, who were mandated to quarantine for 14 days. I recall some debate about this strategy at the time – was this an over-reaction to what may be a mild illness?

As the world received more information from China (via media, publications and the WHO-China joint mission report on Covid-19), it became evident that this virus was a significant threat to humanity. Even with a relatively low case fatality rate, rapid dissemination through a non-immune population creates large absolute numbers of sick patients that can rapidly overwhelm health systems.

The situation escalated rapidly. The weeks that followed were incredibly intense, as healthcare workers globally grappled with an overwhelming volume of rapidly changing information, a deluge of questions and requests from work, colleagues, family, friends, friends of friends…. As a specialist, I am accustomed to assessing and absorbing various sources of information, in order to provide a coherent, evidence-based opinion to colleagues and patients. As the Covid-19 pandemic took off, this process was hyper-charged. My inbox was beset with hundreds of emails per day. Information and opinions flowed rapidly among physicians' networking groups. Within each communication usually lay important pearls. However, the background noise was deafening. Purported findings from pre-print articles were shared widely and became gospel. It felt as though in every clinical workplace, professionals were battling to make the best decisions with limited information. Strongly stated opinions one day quickly looked ridiculous the next in light of new information. I quickly learned to qualify all of my advice with a disclaimer that my opinion could very well change tomorrow as further evidence emerged.

Within the requests for information from colleagues and loved ones sat significant anxiety about what might come to pass. As the pandemic hit Europe and news arose of the terrible death toll in Italy, footage from that region made my blood run cold. The unease around March was palpable as clinicians geared up to metaphorically 'go to war'. Scrubs were dusted off. I was sobered by the logistical discussions on hospital committees relating to allocation of ventilators and palliative care. As New South Wales went into lockdown at the end of March, it felt utterly surreal to suddenly find food shortages, empty shelves and panic buying.

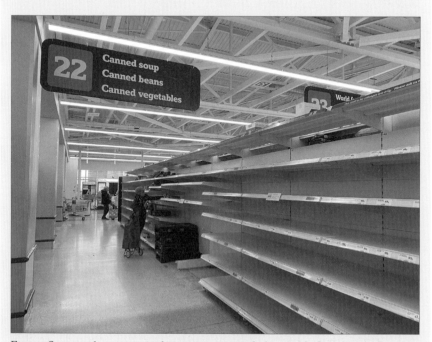

Empty Supermarkets were a phenomenon around the world. Sainsbury's, London, March 18 2020. (*Photo by John Cameron on Unsplash*)

How has the Covid-19 pandemic been managed in Australia? The borders to China were closed early on, and this was subsequently extended to other regions that were deemed high-risk based on emerging epidemiological information. On 20 March, Australian borders to all non-residents were closed and around one week later, enforced hotel quarantine for all arrivals was instituted. These measures, to my mind, have been crucial in pursuing the stated National Cabinet goal of 'zero community transmission'. Restrictions on gatherings were implemented and tailored in response to contemporaneous case numbers. 'Covid-19-safe' advice for businesses was developed and a centralised mandatory check-in system was developed for restaurants and bars open outside of lockdown periods. In Sydney, mask wearing in public indoor settings and public transport is currently mandated.

Our communities have been through lockdowns at various points during the pandemic. In Australia some decisions are made at state and some at federal (national) level. There were widespread lockdown measures between March to May 2020, as well as other more localised lockdown periods between June and October in Victoria, which suffered a significant outbreak at that time. The policies restricting overseas arrivals, mandating hotel quarantine and enforcing lockdown have undoubtedly been an infringement on personal liberty. They have caused economic and emotional distress to many. However, what they have done is buy time. Time to understand the virus. Time to upscale our capabilities. Time to put surge staffing in place. Time to get ahead of the virus, by identifying and quarantining contacts before our contact tracing capacity became overwhelmed. And time to steel ourselves for possible eventualities.

In parallel to restrictions on gathering and movement, there was a surging of the public health workforce. Capacity for community Covid-19 testing was established and upscaled early, alongside strong messaging to the community that they should get tested if symptomatic and then stay at home. Daily public briefings, in which government and health agencies stand side by side, are the norm, delivering unified messages to the community about infection rates and current advice. Every single identified case of Covid-19 provokes a rapid public health response. Finding pre-symptomatic persons is crucial for preventing ongoing transmission. On the outside it looks quiet. Friends that don't work in healthcare comment that 'it must have settled down now for you'. But in the background, an immense amount of effort by a sizeable workforce is required in order to quell each outbreak and keep our case numbers so low.

Clinical services have pivoted to adjust to the pandemic here, as they have done worldwide. Changes include increased use of telehealth, visitor restrictions, rearrangement of wards, innumerable policy meetings, staff screening and a change in culture to ensure those who are sick do not come to work.

The pandemic has stretched healthcare workers – intellectually, emotionally and ethically. There have been robust debates around treatment decisions. These include assessment of limited information and the ethics of giving off label treatments. As I write, the evidence points towards treatment with remdesivir (for some patient groups) and dexamethasone, but this may continue to evolve. I have experienced nosocomial Covid-19 outbreaks in two hospitals. These are complex, time consuming and stressful to manage. In this context, balancing the requirement to isolate potential contacts with the need to continue to safely staff a hospital is extremely challenging. Other contentious clinical discussions have included the type of PPE that should be used, visitor restrictions, maintenance of 'business as usual' activities and how to manage end of life care.

As a Brit living abroad, the UK has never felt further away. For me, 2020's low point was listening to my husband telling his elderly parents that we would probably be unable to return home should the worst happen. We live in a multicultural city and have friends who've lost loved ones and have been not been able to travel to be with their families. As things stand, Australian citizens are required to apply for an exemption to be permitted to leave the country and there is a cap on returning overseas arrivals. Even if these issues are successfully negotiated, organising flights and two weeks in hotel quarantine on return can be challenging and prohibitively expensive. I hope that those we love can keep safe until we see them again. As I write, the UK is experiencing yet another wave and have seen emergence of a variant that appears to be more transmissible. I can see that the pandemic has been managed quite differently in the UK compared to Australia.

The pandemic has been a great amplifier. In workplaces and throughout society, systems and relationships that were already precarious have become more fractious. I worry for my patients who are already experiencing financial hardship, domestic violence or mental illness. Life as a medic with young children has always been intense, but this year everything has been magnified. The relentless march of childcare-associated illness, which has always been tricky to manage, now requires Covid-19 swabs and strict isolation, juggling working from home and guilt at leaving colleagues in the lurch, but wanting to do the right thing. Some days feel impossible.

Conversely, the emergence of SARS-CoV-2 has galvanised healthcare workers and united colleagues in a manner that I have never witnessed before in my career. I have been proud to combine forces with some incredible colleagues as we work together through this challenge. Respectful and collaborative shared decision making (often under very difficult circumstances) has resulted in good outcomes and forged relationships that I hope will last beyond the pandemic. International colleagues have reconnected to pool minds and skills on research projects. We have tested the concept of working from home and (despite its limitations when children are home) may realise the benefits of embracing this in years to come, including less commuter traffic and better access for remote communities to telehealth. Personally, I have reconnected with friends and family. We spend less time in shops and restaurants and more time enjoying nature. New skills have been learned. There have been many silver linings.

I feel very grateful to live in a country that has taken Covid-19 seriously from the outset. Compared to what I have seen elsewhere, it appears that our government and the public have generally listened to scientists and doctors. Health is valued highly in Australia. This approach to tackling Covid-19 has granted us periods of relative normality, during which there is little or no community transmission. During these times it is joyful to be able to attend restaurants and parks with friends. I value these times so much now, though miss the hugs when I greet people.

As 2021 kickstarts, we are watching the incredible efforts that some other countries are making in delivering vaccination programs. Will immunisation provide the exit pass we all wish for from this horrible situation? The data on vaccine efficacy from preliminary phase 2/3 studies looks promising, but we eagerly await further data. Preparations are underway to commence a vaccination program in Australia. Arguably our effective public health response has bought us a little more time to gather information and inform optimal program delivery. Questions remain regarding the duration of protection and whether the vaccines result in sterilising immunity (whether they stop a person carrying and passing on the virus or just from becoming sick). Hand-in-hand with this for Australians comes the question of what the long-term strategy is. Can we achieve herd immunity? And crucially, when will it be safe to reopen our external borders?

Despite incredible developments within a short time period, I expect that it will be some time before this pandemic is over. I hope that as a global community we are able to pull together in an equitable and collaborative manner to get through this, including supporting our most vulnerable society members locally and internationally. Hopefully the skills we have learned will serve us well for our next major existential threat."

Covid-19 on both sides of the pond

Dr Judith McCartney is a Clinical Fellow in Critical Care in Scotland. She was completing her Masters in Public Health at Yale University in America in early 2020 and shares her unique insights into the pandemic.

"When the first wave hit in the UK, I was completing a Masters in Public Health in America. I had left my training as a doctor in anaesthesia in Glasgow, never expecting that when I returned to work the following year, it would be in the midst of a global pandemic. My public health degree could never have felt more relevant or well timed!

I first learned about Covid-19 during a lecture in January. Even then, the full scale of the pandemic didn't personally hit me, until the state went into complete lockdown and flights started to be cancelled from the US to the UK. The thought of being stuck abroad and the gnawing guilt of not working when I knew I could be helping in my local intensive care unit meant I quickly booked my flight home. Flying home on an empty transatlantic flight and arriving back to an almost silent Glasgow airport, really stressed how quickly Covid-19 had grounded normal life as we knew it to a total standstill.

That silence was shattered by my first shift back in the Queen Elizabeth University Hospital Critical Care Unit. While much of the hospital's elective work had been forced to temporarily halt, the Intensive Care Unit was pounding with activity. Scores of extra doctors and nurses had been redeployed to help manage the waves of patients who needed admitting, some with limited experience of working in this very stressful environment. Nurses whose job were usually based in an outpatient clinic were being faced with some of the sickest patients I have ever looked after. While capacity was able to grow, by extending our critical care units across an entire floor of the hospital, our ability to look after more patients, as is typical within the NHS, was principally limited by a lack of staff. Managing an intensive care patient requires specialist skills, not easily acquired quickly or during a pandemic where even the most senior nurses and doctors are struggling.

Personally, I found the first few weeks back on the unit completely overwhelming. The change in pace and pressure from academic and student life; adjusting to the oppressive heat and claustrophobia of the PPE and the sheer mental and physical exhaustion of looking after such unwell patients. I really questioned my decision to return to clinical practice, as I struggled to adjust to the never-ending volume of work and managing patients that seemed to defy all the normal practices of critical care. But like many doctors and nurses who returned to the NHS during this time, knowing you could help in any way, regardless of how small, was enough to convince me, that I had made the right decision.

What I struggled with most during the first wave, and what I still find the most challenging and emotionally draining side of caring for Covid-19 patients, is families not being able to see their loved ones. Only speaking to relatives on the phone will never replace building a relationship with families in person – regardless of how well you hope you are communicating the realities of their relatives' condition. The trauma of missing this time will stay with families for generations. They not only missed the effort of the bedside nurses to care and maintain dignity with simple things like brushing a patient's hair or playing their favourite music, they missed seeing for themselves the really brutal back-aching work of Covid-19 patients: the proning, the management of the inevitable acute deteriorations and the stress and debate between medical teams of how to manage this new disease. I think that is sometimes forgotten in the media narrative. Medical practice is based on evidence, the patterns of learning we develop over years of medical school and up-to-date clinical trials. This was a completely new and terrifying condition, of unknown peaks and troughs. There were no textbooks or studies to rely on, just on-the-job learning. It was a completely new experience for our team.

I always felt that as an organisation, the NHS relies heavily on the strength and goodwill of its staff to deliver care, even when facing staff shortages, funding cuts and ever-increasing clinical demands. During 2020, that goodwill was tested to its very limit. Working long hours, potentially exposing yourself to a deadly virus and managing all this under the scrutiny of the world's media was extremely challenging. While the medical teams managed the patients, the non-clinical staff kept the mechanics of the hospital machine ticking over; the domestic staff, the porters, auxiliary staff restocking our equipment and hospitality staff who made sure we could eat during night shifts, without whom delivering excellent patient care is impossible.

Public support for healthcare workers and the NHS felt highest during the first wave, the collective energy of a nation shocked by the images of patients on ventilators or lying prone, struggling to survive. Now, writing this almost eight months on, this enthusiasm has been subdued, and we are in the midst of the inevitable second wave. As a medical team, we reflected on our management of patients during the first wave and have grown in confidence in managing Covid-19 patients. That doesn't take away the ongoing human cost of this second wave, which I have found almost harder to process than during the first. People are tired, suffering economically and socially isolated and when a vaccine was recently announced, I felt happier than I had felt at any point since this all started. My mum and sisters are doctors too, and the anxiety of all of us working throughout this has been weighing on me every day, especially when my mum, who is in her 60s, faced working as a GP with inadequate PPE. Ultimately, the only way out of this is a large-scale vaccination program and I hope the public trusts, as they have mostly up to this point, the science and the experts in delivering an effective vaccination programme.

Having just spent a year studying American health policy it has been really difficult to watch the challenges America has faced without strong national leadership and a clear strategy to manage Covid-19. Globally, America is one of the wealthiest countries and the failings of their government to contain the virus is down to chronically underfunding public health and a lack of access to universal healthcare and a public health system. Access to healthcare relies on an individual being able to afford appropriate insurance. The NHS was the only line of defence for so many people who contracted Covid-19, where many Americans faced the agonising choice of seeking medical care with its devastating medical bills, or staying home and dying.

What I hope is taken from the horror of 2020 and the Covid-19 pandemic, is that there is no substitute for robust public health infrastructure. This pandemic may have caught many in government off guard, but public health specialists have been warning for years of the devastation that a respiratory pandemic would cause and the need to invest in public health. I hope the efforts and sacrifices of all NHS staff are not forgotten and our national pride in our healthcare is reflected in future health policies. Covid-19 is an opportunity to reset the dial on what is important, with public health being critical to maintaining not only our health, but our economic stability, peace and security."

How Singapore coped with Covid-19

Dr Rebecca Daly is a UK trained GP, who was working in private practice in Singapore when the pandemic hit.

"In 2019, I joined the increasing number of UK trained doctors turning their back on their beloved NHS and I moved with my family to Singapore to work as family doctor in an expat population.

Suddenly, gone are the NHS standard blue walls, carpeted floors and long waiting times for appointments. I now work in the world of private medicine, where my patients are served cappuccinos and cookies in the waiting room. My prescribing practices and referral rates are not at the mercy of a local authority and I can facilitate a same-day specialist appointment for my patient with ease. Undeniably, the medicine is the same; however, I now have the time I need to sit with my patients and provide the holistic care all doctors strive for. I can deliver comprehensive preventative medicine, the backbone of primary care, being able to tailor health screening to the patient's risk factors rather than the national cost-effective programme. A new realisation dawned on me, that I had been rationing medicine through my whole NHS career, where budgets had often hampered clinical care, and treatment decisions were made based on cost per year of life saving.

On the 3 January 2020, I was four months into my new job and still settling into our new life in Singapore when a circular from the Singaporean Ministry of Health landed on my desk warning of a cluster of cases of severe pneumonia of unknown cause in the city of Wuhan, China. A quick Google of Wuhan and a mental note made of the particulars and I started my clinic, unaware that only 20 days later Singapore would see its first case, and even more unthinkable, that in two months' time the World Health Organisation would be announcing a global pandemic of what we now know as Covid-19. The management of this pandemic only highlighted the dichotomy between the healthcare systems of Singapore and the NHS.

Singapore had a head start, as this was not the first pandemic suffered in recent years. Significant lessons had been learnt from the experience of SARS in 2003. Substantial pandemic preparation had occurred – a new National Centre of Infectious Disease had been built and contingency plans for managing PPE and food supplies in the state of a pandemic were drafted. People took it upon themselves to wear masks quite early on and temperature screening and disinfectant handwash were commonplace almost overnight. Within our own clinic, protocols were expedited as soon as the first case was announced in Singapore. To allow safe working practices, patients were screened for symptoms and travel history on the phone and at the clinic door. Patients and doctors undertook temperature screening twice a day. Anyone identified at high risk of Covid-19, were immediately referred for testing as Singapore initiated a rigorous test, isolate and trace policy.

I was supplied with full PPE (including gown, cap, goggles, FFP3 mask and visor), while hearing from colleagues in the UK about their struggles to find scrubs, and of their ingenious ways of sourcing their own equipment from hardware stores, or by relying on donations from local schools for protective goggles. I was even more aghast to hear of doctors being told they were not allowed to wear their own sourced PPE, even though they were only provided with a surgical mask, apron and gloves for any face to face contacts.

In this new Covid-19 world, Singapore's government was better placed to quickly implement measures to control the spread of a pandemic. While I watched escalating statistics of loss of life in the UK, after an earlier plan for herd immunity, Singapore was diligently wearing masks and logging all movements on a tracing app. Only a few days after the first case in Singapore, travel restrictions were implemented, with a two week 'stay at home' notice for returning Singaporeans. Non-adherence to the measures could result in a considerable fine, imprisonment or work visas for foreign nationals being revoked. A comprehensive policy commenced to test symptomatic patients, admit and isolate positive cases and then trace any potential contacts. This required considerable manpower, which came quite literally from an army of people, in the form of the national servicemen of the Singapore Armed Forces.

When my son's teacher tested positive for Covid-19, I experienced the rigour of the Singapore test and trace system first hand. We were notified on the phone of the contact, and visited at the house by an officer from the Ministry of Health to serve our quarantine papers, dictating my son and a primary carer (myself) had to remain isolated in one room of the house until two weeks after the last contact with the positive case. We were supplied with a thermometer and were to expect video calls three times a day to confirm his temperature readings and to prove we were still isolating. We were warned of the possibility of random spot checks at the house and reminded of the disciplinary procedures for non-adherence. We were supplied with two surgical masks, to be used if we needed to travel to the hospital if he became symptomatic. We later received a card from the local community centre, encouraging us to call if we needed any help with groceries or other errands and to wish us good health.

By 24 March, all short-term visitors to Singapore were banned, even if transiting through the airport, and a trace app was in widespread use to help with tracking cases. During the same month in the UK, sporting events and other large-scale gatherings were still permitted. Pubs remained open with the onus on the public not to patronise them, and images of The Stereophonics playing to a crowd of 5,000 in Cardiff were being circulated around the world. The UK decided to adopt a mandatory two-week quarantine period for all travellers to the UK – but not until 22 May. Flights had continued throughout this period, including from affected areas in China.

Despite all this, watching from afar as the Covid-19 story unfolded in the UK, I have never felt so proud of the NHS and all it represents. Staff have shown an incredible ability to adapt and reorganise. I am aware of doctors volunteering to man 111 calls and provide their services to temporary hospitals, such as the Nightingale in London. I have seen primary and secondary care come together, sharing knowledge from their experience at the coalface of the pandemic. The ability to coordinate care on a large scale being demonstrated as doctors were deployed to other specialities and GPs rearranged clinics to be able to provide safe care to their patient communities. The NHS staff were holding up the healthcare of the country despite their lack of PPE, reaching out to those most vulnerable during these challenging times. My hopes for the future of the NHS is that we can learn from this pandemic. Primary care has had to question its delivery of services and consider what is achievable and necessary with limited resources. I am sure the telemedicine revolution will not subside with the end of Covid-19. I also hope the nation has a greater appreciation of the NHS with its finite resources, for it is an envied system that provides healthcare for all, free at the point of care."

(A version of this story first appeared in *The NHS: The Story So Far*)

29 September 2020
Back in the UK, Covid-19 cases are on the rise again. The cooler weather sends people indoors, where the virus spreads more easily and hospital admissions due to the virus have doubled in England over the preceding fortnight. Further restrictions are imposed, including a 10pm curfew for hospitality venues [NHS PROVIDERS 2020]. The global death toll passes 1 million [BFPG 2020].

October

- 34,495,176 cases globally; 1,025,729 deaths
- 460,178 cases in the UK; 42,464 deaths
  (WHO 2020a GOV.UK 2021)

1 October 2020
The Immigration Health Surcharge reimbursement scheme opens to exempt all health and care workers from the fee to access the NHS following their efforts during the pandemic. In May, Boris Johnson was reluctant to scrap this charge, stating the contributions raised £900m for the NHS [NHS PROVIDERS 2020] (see 21 May above).

2 October 2020
Local lockdowns are enforced across the UK, with around 16.8 million people affected [BBC 2020n].

12 October 2020

As cases continue to rise, it transpires that SAGE recommended a short 'circuit breaker' lockdown in September as a way of controlling the virus. The Prime Minister announces a three-tier system of restrictions taking effect from 14 October [BBC 2020o].

Dentistry and Covid-19

Jack Gooding works as a dentist in the North East of England, at a practice providing a mix of both NHS and private dental care. He tells us how the pandemic has negatively impacted dentistry in the UK.

"To limit transmission of Covid-19, dental practices were instructed to close and cease all routine dental care from 25 March 2020. Covid-19 completely shut down the private dental industry from mid-March to early June, while the NHS service was left in chaos trying to pick up the pieces. What the government failed to recognise is that while private

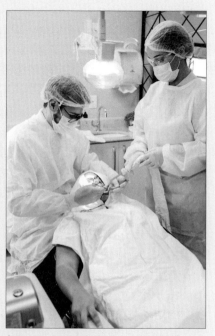

(Photo by Jonathan Borba on Unsplash)

dentists do not work for the NHS, they provide a lot of dental care for the public (due to the fact that there aren't enough NHS practices in some areas), and without them providing this service, the strain on NHS dentistry markedly increases.

While services were suspended, the private dental sector received no financial support from the government and many practices therefore closed. The business owners received some small grants, but it was the dental associates that suffered the most. Many of them were self-employed and normally earning over £50k/year and so received no financial support. Colleagues in this position struggled to get by and relied entirely on their partners income for three months.

Meanwhile, NHS dentistry was in a state of disarray. It was unclear if practices would get any funding or if we would be furloughed or not. After six weeks of uncertainty, the government promised to honour NHS contracts with continued payment, as long as dentists continued to provide patients with remote triage advice, which of course was welcome news.

For the patients, there was no real provision for anyone in dental pain for the first six to eight weeks of the pandemic. During lockdown, we were able to remotely triage patients by phone, but the only help I could offer was 'AAA' – advice, analgesics and antibiotic provision. I couldn't arrange any kind of dental work, be it extraction or otherwise. Unfortunately, there are certain types of dental pain where antibiotics will make no difference whatsoever, and the only relief will be provided by physical intervention such as extraction. Patients were calling me with pain scores of 9–10/10 despite taking painkillers, and I could offer them nothing more.

At our practice we would have one dentist in each day to man the phones. Patients would then knock on the door and we would post our prescriptions through the door as we were unable to remotely prescribe. As dentists, there is not much we can do remotely, it is a job where we are trained specifically to avoid giving antibiotics and aim to physically treat pain to avoid antibiotic resistance. Covid-19 turned this on its head and antibiotics were being prescribed even when there was a chance they would resolve nothing. There was simply nothing we could do and nowhere we could refer to initially. It was a very difficult time and I felt frustrated, helpless and open to complaints. Patients were rightly angry and scared.

By the end of April, the first dental hubs started to open, so we could start to refer for extractions, but it took far too long to get to that point. Patients were frequently going round in circles calling 111 or their GP. 111 could eventually refer to dental hubs when they became operational. The delays were mainly due to a lack of PPE. At the start of lockdown, dental practices had been asked to donate all PPE to hospitals, meaning when dental hubs were needed, no one had the PPE to offer help. Practices were asked to buy in new PPE at overinflated prices at their own cost, which put many off, or meant that many simply couldn't afford to.

Dentists reopened for treatment on 7 June 2020 – we found out about this along with the general public during the Prime Minister's briefing on 4 June. We had no pre-warning internally within the profession and it left little to no time for practices to prepare. Since June, practices have been working to as much capacity as they can, but this is happening at different speeds for different practices – initially due to availability of PPE and now more due to lack of clarity over how practices will be remunerated.

As winter approaches, the situation remains bleak. As of early October, I have a backlog of over 100 patients. I get through three to five a week, but add a further five new patients to my list every week. We are in the minority of NHS practices in that we are actively treating patients who had open courses of treatment before lockdown. Most practices are still seeing emergencies only while their lists grow ever longer.

To understand why this is such a huge problem it is important to realise that, generally, dentists work as quickly as possible due to enforced targets. Five minute appointments are not uncommon. Pre-Covid-19, I would see over 100 patients in an average week in order to meet my targets, so the practice can be paid. Post-Covid-19, we are required to leave one hour fallow time between each appointment to allow particles to settle before a full clean of the surgery takes place. This significantly limits appointments, meaning I can only see between four and seven patients a week plus eight to ten emergencies (which may be unregistered patients). Furthermore, we are mandated to have one surgery room out of use to provide an area to don/doff PPE, and one surgery for seeing emergency patients requiring non-aerosol generating procedures. Any surgeries that don't have ventilation (e.g. a window) cannot be used. So out of our five-surgery practice only one room is seeing patients for routine treatment on a daily basis.

I cannot foresee how we can return to 50 per cent of our normal capacity within the next twelve to eighteen months without the whole system being changed in order to remunerate practices fairly. Who will see the patients we cannot? The future for NHS dentistry is very much in danger.

In the event of a second wave, most practices now have the procedure, protocols and PPE in place to handle emergency dentistry. Hubs will be easier to establish second time around. Routine dentistry will be the hardest hit and private practices will again suffer. The morale within the profession is at an all-time low. Obviously Covid-19 could not have been prevented, but the way that the heads of NHS England, the government and the Chief Dental Officer have handled the pandemic has been confusing, disrespectful and has left many feeling undervalued.

There is a huge amount of anxiety in the NHS sector over how we will ever get back to a sense of normality and whether the service can take the strain of the demand that is building. Retaining dentists to work in the NHS has been a difficult problem over the last few years but it will worsen, with many moving to private dentistry not for financial gain but for reduced stress, more time with patients, and a greater freedom to provide premium quality dentistry. I would hope that the government recognise that it would be better to promote a system that values the quality of the treatment provided rather than the quantity of patients the practice can get through, but my fear is with the backlog as it is and with the fact that there are already millions of people who cannot find an NHS dentist that things will only get worse before they get better."

20 October 2020
The Covid death toll rises by 241, the highest daily increase for months [SIDDIQUE, H 2020]. This figure continues to grow throughout the autumn.

31 October 2020
A second national lockdown for England is announced as the UK passes 1 million confirmed cases. The number of Covid-related hospitalisations hits new highs in fourteen European countries this week [BFPG 2020].

Long Covid

Dr Tracy Briggs, a Senior Clinical Lecturer in Genomic Medicine at The University of Manchester, writes about her experience of Long Covid.

"Until March 2020, I worked full-time as a clinical academic, was a busy mum, commuted to work on my bike and enjoyed rambling and yoga. Then I developed Covid-19.

Despite attending A&E with significant shortness of breath several times during the initial illness, I did not require hospital admission, so I wasn't tested for Covid-19, as was the rule at the time. I was diagnosed with 'mild' Covid-19 since I didn't require admission – although in truth, the 14 days of rigors, night sweats, cough, burning throat, chest pain, palpitations and dysphagia, along with 5kg of weight loss and breathlessness did not feel mild. But of course, I am very grateful to have survived.

I was reviewed 7 days into the illness, at which point I was tachycardic (racing pulse), hypertensive (high blood pressure), lymphopenic (low white blood cells) and hyponatraemic (low sodium levels), but my chest X-ray and other bloods were normal and my oxygen levels remained above 92 per cent. After 14 days things seemed to ease a little and I came out of isolation in my bedroom and met my family again. I continued to feel breathless and have palpitations, but things seemed to be improving until around four weeks later, when the shortness of breath and tachycardia returned with fury. A flight of stairs was a mountain; sitting up to eat a meal at the table – impossible; going out – not an option. I was scared. I was not getting better within a few weeks, like the guidance implied I should, and I thought I was going crazy. At first, I rang work every week to extend my return to work date, but I started to realise this was not realistic.

A few months on, after a normal CTPA (lung scan) and echo (heart scan), I still wasn't getting better. My life had totally changed since having this disease. I spent my time in bed or on the sofa. My husband cooked all the meals, did all the housework and all the childcare. That may sound idyllic, but it was awful. I felt utterly useless. Friends and family would send messages to see if I was recovering, and I wasn't. How was I going to return to work, look after my family, 'be me?'

when I couldn't even hold a conversation or make a cup of tea? Then a friend sent me a newspaper article about Covid patients who have symptoms for months which are 'weird as hell' according to Professor Paul Garner [HARDING, L 2020a]. I realised there were others who didn't need hospital admission who had ongoing symptoms like me, and I cried with relief.

Since then, it has been a long nine months, on a very undulating path. I still have episodes where I end up flat on the floor at the top of stairs with a heart rate of 150 bpm and feel very short of breath. I am not yet back at work and I can do very little around the house.

Living with a condition that is not yet understood, combined with the ongoing restrictions to normal life and normal access to medical care has been difficult. I suffer with ongoing tachycardia and breathlessness and have developed new symptoms of recurrent oral and possible esophageal candidiasis (thrush). I've experienced haemoptysis (coughing up blood) – thankfully only once, acid reflux and chilblains. I have tried to build my own medical management team and plan, which has not been easy with ongoing health issues, but I acknowledge that I am very lucky to have some wonderful, supportive friends and colleagues in medicine, physiotherapy and nutrition to help me navigate. Finding 'the right GP' really changed how I was able to cope with living through this. It is, I now realise, imperative in a condition which seems besieged by set-backs to have someone who listens, supports and, when appropriate, refers on. I know many fellow long-haulers who have been less fortunate and have experienced repeated medical gas lighting and disbelief of symptoms. I have personally been told on two separate occasions that my symptoms are all anxiety related and given that I was PCR negative (a month after onset) and antibody negative (80 days after symptoms) that I have not, in fact, had Covid-19.

I now feel it is vital to increase awareness and understanding of Long Covid, especially to highlight that previously active, young people may not recover after 14 days, as was very much the narrative in the first wave. I was involved in a newspaper article about my experience [HARDING, L. 2020b], and through this I was connected with many others in a similar position. I am now a member of a support group of long-haul UK doctors who have become virtual friends, with whom I have found shared experiences, shared coping strategies and invaluable occupational advice. My networks have also led to the opportunity to take part in research, which is crucial to discover more about this condition. I was appointed community representative for the Covid-19 ACT-Accelerator Therapeutics Pillar, a global initiative whose aim is to save lives and reduce severe Covid-19 disease [WHO 2020c].

I do not know what the future holds for me. Will I get better? Will I get back to work? Will I walk up the stairs again without thinking Ben Nevis was once easier? What will happen if I contract Covid-19 again? I do hope that the recently released Long Covid NICE guidelines [NICE 2020] actually lead to increased care and compassion for all those affected. I hope that clinical services will pull together specialists who can provide the multi-organ follow up that is needed and that this will be accessible throughout the country. I hope that meaningful, individualised rehabilitation will be developed and that patient centred research is undertaken. This seems key for those of us already enduring Long Covid but as the pandemic continues, there will undoubtedly be more. If 10 per cent of those affected with Covid-19 develop Long Covid, as some studies suggest, the medical, economic and social costs are colossal. Certainly personally, living with it, the effects are absolutely devastating."

November

- 45,968,799 cases globally; 1,192,911 deaths
- 1,034,914 cases in the UK; 47,980 deaths
  (WHO 2020a, GOV.UK 2021)

5 November 2020

England's second lockdown begins. In Liverpool, mass-testing begins, aiming to cover all 500,000 people living and working in the city who are willing to come forward. Originally proposed under the name 'Operation Moonshot', the scheme is hailed as a glimpse of an exit strategy, using a combination of PCR swab tests and new lateral flow tests which can rapidly turn around results without being processed in a lab. Success relies on not only detecting those positive for the virus, but convincing them to self-isolate (only 20–25 per cent of people are estimated to comply with quarantine when asked to do so by test and trace) [BOSELEY S et al 2020].

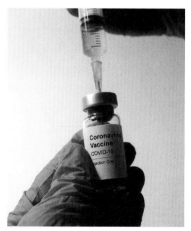

9 November 2020
The Pfizer/BioNTech Covid vaccine is reported to protect 90 per cent of trial recipients [NHS PROVIDERS 2020].

Covid-19 vaccination. (*Photo by Hakan Nural on Unsplash*)

11 November 2020
The UK becomes the first country in Europe to pass 50,000 Covid deaths

The Plague Doctor
Dr Daniel Berkeley is a GP partner in Maryport, Cumbria, and describes how the pandemic affected his rural practice.

"It's the second Thursday morning of March 2020 and I'm sitting in our practice meeting. 'This virus is actually looking pretty bad,' says our senior partner. She is worth listening to. None of us want to hear. We already know. The great thing about GP partnership is the ability to change things quickly, but with that comes a rapidly learnt inertia against changing things 'too soon'.

'We need to cancel everything don't we?'

We all sit for a long time, thinking about what this means. It means everything changes, for our patients, our staff and us.

'Yeah, we do don't we.'

So, we did.

We created one giant telephone surgery list, which would fill up within moments of the phone lines opening, (technically it didn't fill as it was an infinite list!) and we all spent the day phoning back anyone who called us.

As usual our patients amazed us. Rather than panic and try to get onto the list with very minor problems, they left us to deal with the pandemic, for several months at least. But of course, in the end the routine work which forms the bulk of our job had to find a way back in. That's when the real trouble started, but more on that later – in the beginning, we just had the pandemic and emergencies to deal with.

April was the cruellest month. We had no days off. Weekends were a blur of making plans for 'red centres' where we could see Covid-19 positive patients. We got the soldering irons out and reversed the polarity on our surgery ventilation fans to keep viruses in the newly created isolation room. The news coming out of Italy was a spur to us, seeing colleagues falling asleep in corridors and crying as they had to decide which of the three people they had jury-rigged onto one ventilator was going to die. We had to be ready. We thought about death too – death at home. For if the stats were right then we could be facing 300 community deaths in the space of a few weeks in our practice area. The maths showed our four syringe drivers wouldn't be enough. We figured that fentanyl patches, hyoscine patches and buccal midazolam would have to do. I started to think about how these visits would be, it made me think of the medieval plague doctors with their funny hooked beaks full of incense to protect them from the demonic plague. All I had was a flimsy surgical mask. My feeling was that we all have to die one day, and that having survived cancer thirteen years ago at age 23, then I was on borrowed time anyway. I decided I needed armour, so I shaved my head, I'd grow my hair again when this was over.

We watched the 5pm briefing from the Prime Minister every day, watching cases going up and up, but thankfully not in rural Cumbria. Our red hub remained nearly empty, and rapidly our workload went back to dealing with everyday general practice. By June we were the busiest we had ever been, with nearly 200 patients waiting for a call back each day, and very little of it Covid-19 related. I don't blame them – there is only so long you can wait for a routine problem. But the practice didn't feel normal. We were wearing masks constantly; we were stressed and confused and trying to do normal work when things felt far from normal. The usual issues of running a GP practice were back, petty squabbles between staff members, pay demands, car park admin. But the clinical job was completely different, with almost everything done over the phone. Face-to-face appointments were a last resort for problems that couldn't be managed by phone, photo or video. It felt so weird. My little patters had changed, I had now explained how to access therapy via video so many times that it just fell off my tongue (strangely patients were still very adverse to this idea despite it working far better than you might think. I had started psychotherapy myself in February 2020 and had this over Zoom for the vast majority of the pandemic).

By the end of the summer we were all exhausted. The daily triage list had become completely unmanageable, and fuelled by the *Daily Mail*, patients had started to come to the conclusion that we'd not actually been working for the entire year. 'I want this fungal toenail sorted, you've been at home while the hospitals saved us from the pandemic, I don't understand why I can't just come and see you about it.' I didn't argue. There is no point arguing. I just said no and asked for a photo.

Then the second wave came. I write this during the second wave, and things may change, but at present I believe it's clearly going to eclipse the first wave, alongside the added disadvantage of affecting a jaded health system and public.

I caught Covid-19 myself during the second wave. I'd like to say I caught it while heroically seeing a Covid-19 positive patient in an emergency despite a lack of appropriate PPE, but in reality I think I caught it from my wife who caught it from her head of department at school! The first few days were pretty mild – I even worked from home at first, taking great pleasure in being the opposite of what I was being accused by the tabloid press – 'far from taking the year off, I'm working with Covid-19!' But by day three it was clear that I couldn't work. I couldn't breathe, I was being sick constantly and I just couldn't concentrate. My wife and I focused on trying to get better and keep the children safe.

Then, my wife started going purple. She wasn't breathless but I was amazed to find profoundly low oxygen levels when I checked. A modern life plague doctor (paramedic) visited very quickly and whisked her off to hospital. It was midnight and I thought I'd managed to deal with this quietly enough that the children wouldn't know until morning when I could explain properly. Sadly, our middle child had woken during it all and heard, something she didn't tell me for several days.

Trying to explain to three primary school children that their mother is in hospital was even harder than breaking bad news at work, but again, I was struck by their amazing resilience and acceptance. They knew she would get better, and four days later they were right, she came home off oxygen. The real recovery could begin.

Over the course of two weeks all five of our household caught Covid-19 and we received over fifty texts from test and trace and over thirty phone calls telling us we were contacts of people with coronavirus (we were contacts of each other). At one point I cried while trying to get one of the team to let me go so I could care for my children between bouts of being sick – apparently, I had a legal duty to hear his scripted twenty minute speech for a thirtieth time.

For the avoidance of any doubt, 'NHS' test and trace is unutterably broken and would appear to spend most of its funding phoning different family members who've all caught Covid-19 from each other, harassing them. If you want an example of how much trouble the NHS is in, then consider this piece of maths. NHS Test and Trace has so far cost £12 billion – for this we get the shambles I've just described and an 18 per cent rise in the stock value of SERCO, who got a significant chunk of this funding. In return, we as GPs have been asked to vaccinate the entire country against Covid-19 when the vaccine is available, with one eighth of the budget allocated to test and trace (£150 million). Consider for yourself which initiative is more useful. Once again, general practice is significantly undervalued and underfunded.

There is more pandemic to come, but that is a story as yet unwritten. I am left reflecting on the cost so far. The cost to general practice is huge. It's long been the case that the funding system for primary care is not fit for purpose. It was set at a time when on average a patient consulted twice a year, they now consult on average six times a year. General practice receives less than 10 percent of the funding that goes to the NHS, yet does over 90 per cent of the clinical contacts that occur in the NHS. How does this add up? Well, it doesn't – it works on the partnership model where GPs own and run their own practices and therefore work at risk on their profits in lieu of a salary. The only way it works is that we do lots of other things on the side that make enough profit to keep our surgeries running, services like minor surgery, contraceptive implants, STI clinics, HGV medicals – things we had to stop doing due to Covid-19. This is a cost some bigger practices will be able to cover through lean years for the GPs. Smaller practices will disappear and their GPs will go bankrupt without government support.

Then there is the cost to the patient-doctor relationship. Large sections of the press have decided that we have been sitting at home doing nothing, which is far from the reality in that we have helped fight the pandemic at great financial and personal cost. Even when most don't believe this, the effect on morale is huge.

There is the cost to our team as well. We are a big team and we like to reward our staff with parties and a generally fun atmosphere. A year of wearing masks, minimal staff mixing, stress, and no socialising has

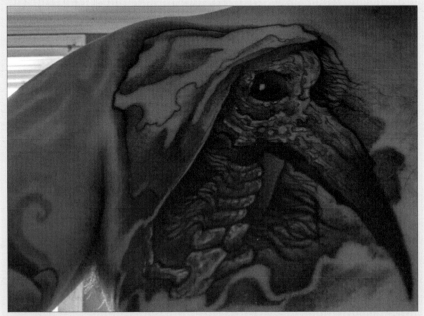

The Plague Doctor Tattoo.

hit morale hard and I continue to worry that we will make it through this as a team fully unscathed.

The cost to the patients is the biggest though. We have had a few Covid-19 deaths, and these are awful, but these are nothing when compared to the morbidity in terms of other physical and mental health. Humans did not evolve to sit at home on their own. This year is destroying the physical and mental health of our patients, and its repercussions will be felt for decades to come.

So, what of the future? We do what we are best at. We keep going. We are the one part of the NHS which cannot run a financial deficit (we are small businesses). We cannot close or transfer our work, and we cannot discharge patients. We just keep going and find a way, we always find a way. We are general practice.

And what of the plague doctor? I now wear him on my chest thanks to my talented tattoo artist."

17 November 2020

The National Audit Office reports that suppliers of PPE with political connections were ten times more likely to be awarded contracts during the pandemic [READ, S 2020].

23 November 2020

Oxford University's AstraZeneca vaccine is reported to be 70 per cent effective, with scientist believing this can rise to 90 per cent with dosing alterations. The government announces its three-tier system for Covid restrictions for the winter [NHS PROVIDERS 2020].

NHS Test and Trace
This piece is written by an anonymous Environmental Health Officer who was drafted in to assist with NHS Test and Trace.

"I have always worked primarily in food safety and health and safety in my role as an Environmental Health Officer, but public health work has always been a key part of our work. Our role in the 1900s was of course as sanitary inspectors, and we play a prime function in the prevention of infectious disease such as E. coli 0157 outbreaks, plus many other bacterial and viral infections.

My team was involved with Covid-19 from the get go, initially providing the businesses we work with, with education and advice on closure and obtaining grants for financial support. Our local test and trace (T&T) work really got going in the summer. We work for the local authorities and pre-Covid also worked alongside PHE dealing with outbreaks and cases of infectious disease – such as norovirus in care homes and nurseries. All of the food and environmental sampling we conduct is done via PHE labs. So our normal role in outbreak management came into play during the pandemic. We received IT training on the local T&T case system and half of our team focused on this, while the other half continued our work ensuring businesses were complying with the Covid-19 regulations and enforcing this where necessary. As things became busier, other county councils and agencies were brought in to assist – and we needed this manpower for enforcement activities!

Our region initially had very few cases of Covid, and when cases were low, we saw the local T&T as an effective system. We know all our businesses very well, so when contacted by workplaces with symptomatic staff, we knew their set up and working practices so knew who to isolate quicker than the national T&T teams, but this became more difficult to manage as cases rose exponentially. Contact tracing for Covid-19 was all done using a computer system from the council. All the cases for the area would go onto the system, then we individually went through the positive cases one by one. We would ring them, gather information about their household, workplace and social contacts and ask them where they had been. If they worked for large employers we needed to get in there quickly and isolate people. Cases like this led to a fast increase in cases locally and many workplaces were not clear on definitions of what it means to be a close contact of a Covid case.

One call to one person could result in twenty further calls – for example if they worked in an office with twenty others with poor air circulation. Some workplaces were conducting their own lateral flow tests, but this could also bring up new cases if asymptomatic people then tested positive. We would look at when symptoms started and look at all contacts 2–3 days before to determine who should be isolated. We often found in the summer transmission occurred 3–5 days prior to symptoms starting. People thought they were doing well socialising outside, but we had cases from BBQ gatherings where people were sharing cutlery and glasses.

In the summer we came across large groups (particularly males) who had been out and about together socially. We would often see a group of five that met together in one pub, but then when they moved onto the next pub, socialised with a group of five different people.

One man had been out drinking in town on four consecutive nights, socialising with hundreds of different people. From that one person there was forty positive cases (and probably, ultimately, many many more).

In autumn I was part of an outbreak control team in schools. We looked at individual school cases and if one positive contact was found then that entire class bubble would be required to isolate. We would then have to look at their other contacts such as breakfast clubs, after school clubs, who they ate lunch with and played with at break times. School buses were a prime place for Covid to be spread. By Christmas we were seeing a lot of transmission in both secondary schools and primary schools. It is likely the new variant was around by then and causing increasing numbers of cases.

I found the Christmas period the hardest, as people were becoming very emotive and the majority had decided they were going to mix with others no matter what their circumstances. We spent a lot of time at T&T being sworn at and having phones slammed down!

My normal job as a food officer inspecting food businesses and awarding food hygiene ratings hasn't been done in person for a year now. Some remote inspections have been possible but not many. Working from home during lockdown and the second round of home schooling was challenging. My son started school in September 2019 and has had a rocky start to his education. My daughter is massively affected by no social contact with friends – the pressure this time round is huge and it's forced me to take time out of work to concentrate on home schooling them. Lockdown itself with everyone at home all the time also has its own challenges!"

December

- 61,866,635 cases globally; 1,448,990 deaths
- 1,643,086 cases in the UK; 60,828 deaths
  (WHO 2020a, GOV.UK 2021)

2 December 2020
The Pfizer/BioNTech vaccine is approved by the Medicines and Healthcare products regulatory Agency, making the UK first in the world to approve a Covid vaccine [MAHASE, E 2020].

8 December 2020
90-year-old Margaret Keenan becomes the first person to receive a Covid vaccine outside of a clinical trial as the vaccination programme is rolled out.

The Vaccine Roll-out (GP Perspective)

Dr Elizabeth Toberty is a salaried GP in Newcastle-Upon-Tyne. She wrote a similar piece in December 2020 for the Huffington Post, *just prior to the launch of the Covid-19 vaccination programme*

"As the first ecstatic news reports arrived announcing the vaccine that we had been eagerly waiting for had arrived, instead of sharing the hope and optimism projected by the media, I had a distinct feeling of unease. Once again, I heard uninformed politicians overpromising that the 'NHS was on standby to deliver'. The knot in my stomach grew stronger as I listened, thinking to myself: 'No we're not'.

Each year general practice rolls out a huge influenza programme. Vaccines are ordered in January and patients get booked in from

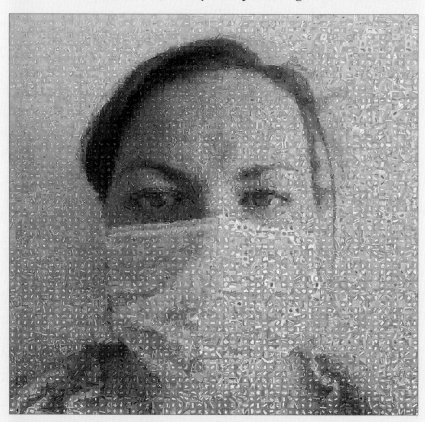

This image of Dr Toberty in PPE was created by Alastair Cross at PicUp. @picupglobal is an environmental community project creating art from documented litter and empowering our communities to discover that each small action contributes to the bigger picture. Find out more: https://www.picup.org.uk

September onwards, even though they're unlikely to catch flu until around Christmas at the earliest. Each surgery has this rehearsed, like a finely oiled machine. Practice managers coordinate it, practice nurses deliver it. And herein lies the magic and power of general practice – we KNOW our patients. It is so poorly understood by policy makers that it rarely features in the reams of waffle pumped out by Whitehall each year. We know how to communicate best with our communities, to just get stuff done. We know this because we have been doing it day in, day out for decades, meaning we know how to organise a flu clinic to result in the highest uptake of a vaccine in our individual population.

And this is why it grates, to have constantly changing, last-minute orders from NHS England. 'Vaccines must be delivered from 8am til 8pm, 7 days a week.' 'Practices must work with their networks and will only receive the payment once both vaccines are given.' 'This vaccine should take priority over routine work.' We are actively depriving general practice of its autonomy, it's magic, the thing that could make this all work.

The specifications for this roll-out have been released to GPs late in the evening, still containing tracked changes and requiring a response within 1–2 working days. It gives the impression of chaos at the top, which does not inspire confidence in a smooth roll-out on the ground.

Coordinating a worldwide first of this nature is an unenviable task but despite it being an evolving situation, NHSE needs to recognise that an efficient roll-out will not be achieved by keeping GPs in the dark. It is unacceptable to release key specifics of the programme to GPs (to enable them to decide if they can participate) while simultaneously running a press narrative that all GP surgeries are ready to go from 14 December. This is simply not true.

Primary care staff will once again suffer the brunt of poor planning and execution from the Department of Health and NHSE. At best we have an extremely difficult logistical task; at worst a recipe for wastage of this precious vaccine, a loss of public confidence and no doubt a huge amount of blame directed towards general practice.

Many GPs have huge reservations around the feasibility of the programme and may not sign up to deliver the vaccine – mainly because the arrangements for their patients are still unclear. As someone on the ground, I can tell you this will result in thousands of patients phoning their practices on Monday morning, potentially blocking the lines for other ill patients. Patients will get frustrated and vent to our already fatigued reception staff, but most concerningly, they may lose confidence in the vaccine itself.

Combine this with directives to halt routine work to prioritise the vaccine, and chaos ensues. GPs know that as soon as routine work stops, urgent, unplanned demand rises – manifesting as unmanageable on-calls for doctors and high A&E attendances. It is not a long-term strategy for delivering this vaccine.

GPs do more than dish out painkillers for arthritic knees. We improve the long-term health of our patients. No one will notice if blood pressures, diabetes and cholesterols are not actively managed for a year or two. But to ignore them is increasing the risk of strokes, heart attacks and possibly cancer. Life expectancy has stalled in our country. If we stop our routine work, deaths will rise from other causes.

Now is not the time for a full overhaul of general practice. But what's making delivering the vaccine harder is the total lack of investment and understanding of what GP is about. Ask general practice what it needs to do this and then deliver the resources necessary, rather than trying to dictate it centrally. Given the eye-watering sums paid to the private sector to deliver track and trace and the like, I suspect the government will be pleasantly surprised what good value for money primary care can offer.

The decision that those over 80 should be first in line for the vaccine ahead of the staff administering the vaccines defies logic. A third of people are asymptomatic from Covid-19. An estimated 1 in 100 people have it, meaning there is a reasonable chance some vaccinators will have, and pass on, the very condition they are vaccinating against. Logic dictates we vaccinate the vaccinators first remembering the old adage: first, do no harm.

Next year, when we are all hopefully vaccinated, we need a stronger, more united primary care, clear about the quality of care we want to bring to our communities. When the latest policy is drafted and it isn't right or appropriate, we must be able to say 'No', without fear of retribution, or a tweet from an inflammatory journalist. We need to be clear we are a finite resource, and to the disappointment of many of our patients, we are only able to provide what they need and not everything they want."

Three months into the vaccination rollout, Dr Toberty tells us her thoughts:

My early jitters about vaccine delivery did not come to fruition. There was confusion, difficulty, and frustration in the early days. However, the sheer desire and determination from primary care staff on the ground to get this programme delivered meant many obstacles were quickly overcome.

Primary care rose, and continues to rise, to the challenge spectacularly. This achievement was driven by the desire to do the right thing for our patients. The success of the programme was partly due to adequate procurement of the vaccines, but mainly because vaccination delivery was devolved to a local level. As GPs, we know our patients – we can contact them easily and they trust us.

The sudden decision by the chief medical officers to delay the second vaccine from three to twelve weeks on New Years Eve, was very poorly communicated and thought out. It caused no end of stress and confusion, and little was done to understand or address the concerns of frontline staff.

I still have worries that general practice will not be adequately remunerated for vaccine delivery, with some areas left financially vulnerable, despite doing this most vital work. I am also still concerned that we are not doing the rest of the important preventative medicine we should be. If there is no intervention to address this in the coming year the knock-on effects will be felt for years to come, likely in the form of widening health inequalities and a lowering of life expectancy.

We need to be confident in how vital general practice is to the health of this nation. No private company could ever replicate the knowledge, skills and care GPs can, and do, provide. No private company could have delivered the vaccine as quickly and efficiently in such a short timescale. We need to speak up and demand the funding necessary to deliver proper primary care if we are to ensure the sustainability of community medicine.

If this vaccination programme has taught us anything, it is to value ourselves, our skills, our intimate understanding of our patient population, and to use our collective voice powerfully in the future to advocate for our patients and the NHS.

The Vaccine Roll-out (Vaccinator Perspective)

Jane Russell spent most of 2020 working as Chief Nurse onboard a cruise ship. When she returned to the UK, the Covid-19 vaccine programme was being rolled out and she got involved as a vaccinator.

"I spent eight-and-a-half months of 2020 stuck on a cruise ship, working as chief nurse, with no shore leave. We had been dealing with an outbreak of Covid-19 so my vacation was very welcome. Two weeks self-isolation in my small Somerset house in mid-November, talking to no one was now in my head equivalent to two weeks on a Barbados beach with an open bar run by Brad Pitt.

Then I got bored…. Normally after a couple of weeks back home I would do a few agency nursing shifts a week, for something to do, a little money and some experience doing 'real' nursing back in the NHS. The thought of jumping into full PPE still filled me with dread after living in it onboard, and my vacation would be over by February. During my self-isolation, news of the vaccine programme was ramping up and I thought it would be ideal for me as the patients would be healthy and happy, it would involve only minimal PPE and my nearest centre was just six miles away.

I contacted the hospital bank and had a telephone interview. I then did four hours online training on Covid-19 and the Pfizer/BioNTech

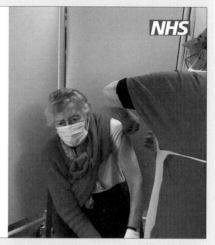

#COVIDvaccine

"I'm so pleased to be one of the first people in the world to receive this vaccine! I hope everyone will take the opportunity to get vaccinated when it is offered to them, so we can start getting back to normal and put this pandemic behind us."

Jean Cook, Somerset's first patient vaccinated against COVID-19

Jane vaccinating Somerset's first patient Jean Cook (shared with permission). (*Yeovil Hospital comms dept*)

Covid-19 vaccine and attended an anaphylaxis and Basic Life Support refresher course.

We started on 8 December. The PGD (Patient Group Directive – a legal framework which allows medication/vaccines to be given without a prescription/directions from a prescriber) wasn't quite ready so after a three to five minute assessment by a nurse, each person had then to see a doctor or nurse prescriber to prescribe the vaccine, and then another nurse to administer the vaccine, they then sat in a room watched by a medical student or HCA for fifteen minutes before leaving. In that fifteen minutes, admin staff would book their appointment for the second dose of the vaccine. Social distancing and creating a workflow were a challenge. The clinic was based in a medical academy which, despite being quiet, was still trying to function around our clinic. The PGD was eventually approved which streamlined the process, and we had two staff from the pharmacy department mixing and drawing up vaccines to match patient flow. We started with fifty the first day and got up to an average of 300 a day, although one day there was a refrigeration glitch and so we did 750. Not one vaccine was wasted.

Appointments were made by a small group of cheerful admin staff pulled from all over the trust, like all of us, doing a new ever-changing job to match the latest government guidelines. As we were one of the first clinics to start in the area, nurses from other Trusts came to see how we had got up and running. Some were going to run clinics in community halls or showgrounds and wanted to follow our organisation of patient flow.

While we only met each patient for two or three minutes, we saw such a mix of emotions. The over 80s mostly very matter-of-fact, unsure of all the fuss but missing grandchildren very much. Anxiety and tears from the needle-phobic were fairly common, and the competition among nursing staff to hear 'Oh, I didn't even feel it,' was real!! One patient, a nurse from an acute area, had been shielding since March, and cried with relief at being a step nearer to returning to the work that she missed very much despite her own health problems.

While it was simple 'conveyor belt' nursing, two things struck me. Obviously it was different to have perfectly healthy 'patients', but

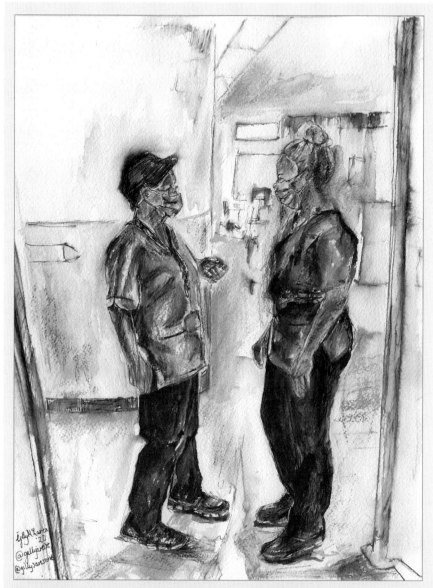

'The Bond of Work Friends – Portraits and Tales from a Hospital Bed'.
(*By @gillyartist with prints available from www.gillyartist.com*)

although there were some concerns about the vaccine that we managed to allay in all but one case, every single person was just so genuinely, humbly thankful, and they were positive that each vaccine was a step toward a return to normal life. Secondly, was our vaccine team – a mixture of bank nurses, matrons from the units drafted in to help for odd days and many retired nurses who rejoined the nurse bank to help. I suspect that most days there was more combined nursing experience in the vaccine clinic than in ED or ICU! I have twenty years' experience in cruise ship medicine. We had an army midwife; a retiree from the resuscitation council; ophthalmic; paediatric; ICU; ED; community nurses – all specialities attended at some point.

I've finished working now to avoid the high-risk area before returning to my other job, but if they're still functioning in the summer when I get my next two months' vacation, I'll be back like a shot … in the upper deltoid."

Health journalism during the Covid crisis
Ellie Philpotts is a features journalist with GP magazine Pulse and winner of awards for 'Best Scoop' award at the British Society of Magazine Editors Talent Awards for her world exclusive on the UK's Covid vaccination programme launch, and 'Best Editorial Assistant'. She describes the realities of being a shielding journalist through the pandemic.

"In journalism, you never really know what's lurking round the corner. Much of the time, the issues of the hour are hard to decipher, and even harder to predict. The news agenda, while often built on a foundation of context, sheds its skin like a snake, replacing in one fell swoop the one it succeeded.

Crystal balls aren't part of a journalist's kit. Instead, our kits include Dictaphones and notebooks, and our profession is based around speaking to people – which should be done whenever possible – collating perspectives like pebbles on a beach (and, if you're a news writer, avoiding whimsical similes…)

You're also meant to be honest about what you don't understand, all while trying to increase how much you do.

Never has this rulebook come into focus, been re-evaluated, and, in some cases, discarded entirely than in 2020, when a novel virus became a little dot on our collective horizons, creeping first into the background of our lives, before sweeping into a once-in-a-lifetime pandemic that took over the world.

I write this in late summer 2021, and the endlessly regenerating cycle hasn't showed much sign of slowing down.

There is no one who remains untouched by Covid-19 in some capacity, and while journalism doubles as a platform for absorbing as many of these takes, my contribution to this book is about a perspective that journalists rightly don't explore so often – their own.

So here is my personal and professional fusion of covering Covid-19 and being enveloped within it, as we all were and still are in our own ways.

2020 began as normal, and so did journalism – as far as it can. Fast-moving news cycles long predate the pandemic, but my stories back then tended to fit the 'standard' mould.

I began as the features assistant at *Pulse*, the leading trade publication for GPs, the year prior. This meant commissioning, editing and managing Continuing Professional Development (CPD) modules, Working Life recounts, case studies, debates, regular bloggers and guest opinion pieces in the monthly print magazine and constantly updated website, while contributing elsewhere in the brand, such as running its social media and firing off an interview here and there.

Despite being interested in it, the nature of my priorities meant it was rare for me to chip into news, although features always had some degree of crossover. Rather, it was my colleagues with titles like 'reporter' and 'news editor' who kept abreast of what GPs needed to know in their daily practice. Aspects such as the recent formation of primary care networks; CQC inspections; CCG board papers; semi-scandalous RCGP council meetings; clinical updates on common drugs; outrages over issues like bureaucracy; and guidance changes.

As well as outputting a daily combination of 'lead' and 'web' stories, *Pulse* has spent its sixty-plus years in business dishing up in-depth analyses and delving into investigations, such as practice closures disproportionately targeting smaller sites and disadvantaged pockets of the country; workload being dumped by secondary care; and, unfortunately, systemic racism manifesting in outcomes like exam results.

By the February, however, no investigation was needed to decipher that something strange was coming, finding its way to land with force on our keyboards and climbing higher and higher up in our articles. It might have started with a small operational shift, or a Public Health update to be fleetingly aware of, about travel through a particular part of China. But its relevance grew and mentions of the virus and its far-reaching implications got closer to the crux of the headlines.

It became clear that news was going to be significantly more important, and there was going to be a lot of it. Of course, there is never a good time for a pandemic, for far more pressing reasons than a magazine's structure, but from a *Pulse*-specific perspective, it started to strike just when we had lost our senior reporter, with our news editor on her final month of maternity leave.

So, I moved over to the newsdesk to give my full attention to reporting. It was a task that needed my full attention. It could be hard to keep up with the rapidly evolving pace – but we knew we had to, and to do it well. GPs genuinely sought out *Pulse* for knowledge of how they should be adapting to the situations conjured up, delivering safe care to a distressed population, while maintaining their place at the forefront of patient interactions. All of this, while trying to protect their own physical and mental health, and their families', as far as they could. GPs have traditionally occupied the seat of the public's first and often most accessible port of call for the whole scope of healthcare needs, and in the urgency of this crisis, that was only exemplified.

What we covered – and still do – varied as much as the messages often did themselves. Sometimes, it was as 'simple' as regurgitating letters to the workforce on standard operating procedures from ruling organisations – which wasn't actually simple at all. Translating content into something understandable was also a major role. Despite GPs being medically-trained whereas our team isn't, and *Pulse* not being intended for members of the public we were often producing content on the crisis that no one, whether NHS England, GPs or political leaders, had lent much imagination to, let alone lived out, before.

The main unions and representative bodies always had something to say too, but, most importantly for us, so did the GPs who form the UK's biggest medical specialty. Their many thousands incorporated all nations of the UK; grassroots; leaders whether on local committees or sitting nationally; and then partners; locums; salaried; portfolio; part-time (who are never really 'part-time'); trainees and every other type of GP you can imagine.

Talking to them – while suddenly no longer in person – is what makes the job what it is. Even more of an honour is having GPs return to you on the back of this, trusting you to convey their experiences with accuracy and flair. Whether they come armed with good intentions and story ideas that ultimately didn't end up as tangible stories; scandals that ended up splashed across the national press; or just snippets of irritations they rightly want to vent, knowing that GPs trust you as their outlet has a lot of meaning.

Finding out how things were progressing or unravelling the ground; the scale of the abuse faced by primary care teams who became undeserving outlets to mounting yet uncontrollable frustrations; and their small wins and assortment of anecdotes of kindness is a crucial part of *Pulse*'s ethos, and an example of a crucial part of being a journalist. This has always been my favourite part of the job, but in the context of a dreadful pandemic, it morphs into the pinnacle of a privilege.

GPs are shouldering the toughest times of their careers, the level of which could never have been hinted at even by their in-depth training. Juggling management of the coalface is far from the full works – alongside Covid-19 itself and all the protocols and anxiety it brings, there are also the many societal branches that their non-clinical duty of care extends to, plus the immense backlog elsewhere.

Through no fault of its own, the NHS was effectively consumed with Covid-19, meaning the postponement of routine surgeries; general practice switching almost overnight to a largely remote triage model; and primary care having to cope with even more pertinent staffing gaps on the back of widespread illness and enforced isolation. The pressure on the system was creaking in a way it never had since its creation in 1948.

Having a role amid the minutiae of general practice's unforeseen challenges – albeit from the comfort of a safe distance, comparatively protected at home – is something I'll always treasure.

Why are GP practices still working differently?

NHS
Greater Glasgow and Clyde

If the pandemic is over why can't I book a face to face GP appointment?

The pandemic is not over.

GP practices are open but are working differently in order to protect patients and staff.

In order to protect the most clinically vulnerable people who are in contact with our health services, some physical distancing requirements remain in place.

How are practices working now?

Most practices are using a "Telephone First" service.

This allows the team to assess patients over the phone and consider who needs to be seen in person and when a telephone consultation or video may be appropriate. This helps to ensure that everyone gets the type of appointment they need, and that people don't have to travel to the surgery if they don't need to.

In many cases the issue can be as effectively managed with a telephone consultation rather than a face to face meeting.

If you need to attend the practice for examination you will be given an appointment.

Why do reception staff ask personal questions?

GP reception staff are vital members of the practice team and treat all information as confidential.

They ask questions to ensure that patients are directed to the best support, within and outwith the practice.

They are trained to ensure patients are seen by the most appropriate member of the practice team and ensure GPs can prioritise the patients with the greatest clinical need.

Why am I seeing someone who is not my GP?

Many GP practices have teams of specialists working alongside the GPs.

These teams have widened and may include Nurses, Health Care Assistants, Advanced Nurse Practitioners, Pharmacists, Physiotherapists, Mental Health workers and Community Links workers.

Your needs may be dealt with more effectively by one of these team members.

Where else can I get help?

NHS Inform (www.nhsinform.scot) has lots of information to help you to help yourself.

Community Pharmacists can help with many common illnesses and can prescribe some medications.

Community Optometrists will advise people with urgent eye complaints.

Community Dentists will manage any dental problems.

What about emergencies?

If you have an urgent health issue please contact your GP practice during the day.

If you have an urgent issue and think you need to go to the Emergency Department please call NHS 24 on 111, day or night.

If you have a life-threatening emergency please **call 999** or go to your local **Emergency Department**.

Please be patient. Please be kind

All our health services are under enormous pressure and our staff are working extremely hard. We are open and here if needed. Please work with us to help us ensure you get the right care, in the right place and at the right time by the appropriate health professional for your needs.

Please treat those who are trying to help you with respect and kindness.

An NHS poster explaining new ways of GP working during the pandemic. (*Reproduced with permission from NHS Greater Glasgow and Clyde*)

Last year threw me into a ferocious news agenda, dominated by just one story. In my first full year as a health journalist, it was a sure-fire way of bidding farewell to the comfort zone I had, without meaning to, tried to curate. There was no chance to look back. As I gained confidence, backed up by my editors' mentorship, I achieved some splashes that made their way to their nationals. One was my world exclusive that the UK's Covid vaccination programme was to launch, with details of its GP-led delivery, at a moment in history when no vaccines had even been approved [KAFFASH, J., PHILPOTTS, E., 2020].

It stemmed from an aspect of journalism that I touched on above and that shouldn't be overlooked – a tip from a contact who remembered me from previously taking the time to speak to them, and won me Best Scoop at the prestigious British Society of Magazine Editors Talent Awards [PULSE 2021a]. I was also named Best Editorial Assistant at this (still virtual!) ceremony, in a much-appreciated nod to how I'd kept the features side ticking away too.

It's poignant to remember that the government instruction to work from home reached teams of all types, the City of London where *Pulse* is usually based amid the bustle became not very bustling at all – the same being true of our own office. Previously, there had been a bit of a joke that the longest I had gone without chatting to my colleagues was twenty minutes, so the move to a solo environment meant I missed them and all of our (very!) regular conversations a lot. Our WhatsApp group and email inboxes were straining under the weight of all the queries and updates, but it was no longer hygienic to chat over the old-school water cooler or morning coffee, usually about topics with the most tenuous connection to work. The strength of our team, though, makes itself known in different ways – the fact that we're still such good friends, as well as close-knit colleagues.

Away from the physical spread of the virus, and isolation being mandated, it's been a people-focused pandemic. Perhaps we have become more connected than before. It's easy to let your job become your identity and entire routine, especially with home working dissolving boundaries by seeing you still typing well into the evening. While often born of a hunger to achieve, it was also because, in all honesty, there wasn't much else to do. With legal sanctions on staying in, and meet-ups and entertainment venues full of life relegated to mere memory, it made sense from a career angle to plough efforts into securing a reliable reputation as a new reporter.

But with burnout rife across industries – and perhaps no more so than in frontline health and social care – that we're all people behind our titles has rarely been more relevant.

As a young person and not just a journalist, I explored the health implications of the pandemic too. To my surprise, I was put onto the 'clinically extremely vulnerable' list that we so often covered, in a clash of worlds.

Correspondences from the Department of Health and Social Care and NHS England landed on my doormat advising me to 'shield' pretty much from the offset. They checked in throughout; reminded me of changing regulations and the need for maintained vigilance; and, more recently, saw me receiving my vaccine doses – in February and April – far ahead of other 25 year olds.

While I'm fortunate to live a conventionally healthy life now, all of this was on the basis of having Hodgkins Lymphoma as a teenager. I probably wouldn't have envisioned when 15 and newly diagnosed with blood cancer that exactly a decade on, I would be spending significant periods in another form of isolation thanks to the threat of another illness beginning with C. But I also wouldn't have imagined that this time, the whole world would effectively be with me, nor how I or anyone else would have responded.

There is also a sadness that reaches far beyond all the professional headlines you're coming up with, and into a personal side instead. I took on the task of managing all of the obituaries and tributes for the GPs who died with Covid – there are, at time of writing, sixteen [PULSE 2020b]. Hearing from their grieving families and colleagues, while trying to do justice to their stories and diverse lives that spanned well beyond their work in general practice or the pandemic, was a privilege on a human level.

At the eager-to-learn start of your career, it's hard to feel jaded, but I don't think this would happen even longer in health journalism either. As it's the speciality I want to stay in, I already think about how burnt out may emerge in time, or even fatigue hearing about medical revelations that should be universally exciting, but, maybe naively, I imagine it to be difficult to become desensitised when the human stories we are told, remain so powerful.

Pulse's good friend and long-term blogger Professor Kailash Chand also died during the pandemic, of non-Covid reasons [Philpotts, E., 2021]. I had spoken to him as usual on the day of his untimely death, and he remains sorely missed by us all. He had been a supporter of *Pulse* for decades, one of my most reliable contacts from as soon as I started, and an unwavering presence as the unpredictability unfolded.

Overall, the pandemic period has been a steep learning curve, but it's been a genuine honour, to act as a health journalist during this period of crisis. It saw trade media receive more of the attention it always should have. While much of the mainstream media lost many GPs as readers thanks to peddling misinterpretations of reality or sustained attacks on the profession who were just doing as instructed – such as on face-to-face access – they have come to rely on publications like *Pulse* even more [PULSE 2021b]. This was evidenced in us gaining a higher readership than the *BMJ* and the *British Journal of General Practice*, according to this year's GP Media Survey [COGORA 2021].

The blend of breaking news, landing exclusives, interviewing GPs and shining the spotlight on doctors still completing valuable and fascinating projects away from the pandemic realm, some working as far afield as Nepal [PULSE 2021c], the Arctic [PULSE 2021d] and Zambia [PULSE 2021e] – has certainly immersed me in all aspects of general practice journalism.

It's renewed my ambition to one day publish my own book based around helping other teenagers confronted with a lonely cancer diagnosis as I was, and restored any slightly waning faith I might have had in the power of both kindness and humanity.

It's been a pandemic of mass tragedy and suffering, here in the UK and much further from home. But the earth is home to us all, and we can all often find another home within words. Words jumped off screens and pages during the time of Covid, offering a supportive touch when touch in its normal format wasn't permitted; advice to the scared, newly hospitalised patient, bereaved partner, or person stuck with the illness in their home; or a flash of hope in the form of the arrival and implementation of the vaccination programme, or survivors' stories. It was and is powerful to have played some small role in all of that."

Conclusion – How the NHS Coped

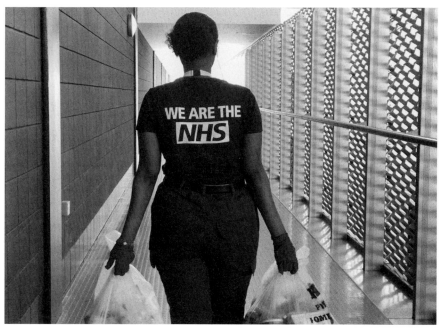

'We are the NHS' taken at The NHS Nightingale Hospital. (*Alex Kumar, Global Health Photography* ©)

The stories in this book have been written in a staggered timeline. Most were told at the peak of the pandemic, in the midst of the action, others from a more reflective position a year on. As the book goes to the final stage of editing, it's autumn 2021 and another gloomy winter is approaching. Britain's Covid infection rate continues to top the league tables as one of the worst in the world [HOWIE, M., 2021]. Masks have been discarded by many; employees are returning to their workplaces and travel restrictions lifting as the country wills itself to return to 'normal'.

Yet normality for the staff of the NHS, bruised and battered from over a year-and-a-half of dealing with this crisis, is that this virus is not going away. Younger, unvaccinated people are being admitted to hospitals [SKY 2021]; GPs are delivering almost 2 million more appointments per month than they were pre-pandemic, while still being accused of being closed by some sections of the media [NHS DIGITAL 2021] and more than 5.45 million people are waiting for hospital treatment in England [BBC 2021a]. The prospect of another winter like that of 2020, or worse, may be enough to finally break NHS staff.

The main difference between a bad situation and a good one is people, and the staff of the NHS and social care services are its greatest asset. This was fully demonstrated during the pandemic. Reports circulated of social care staff moving in with residents during lockdown to prevent an outbreak [BBC 2021b]; GPs fashioning their own PPE to enable them to see patients safely [PULSE 2020], and former NHS staff returning to the frontlines to fight the virus [GMC 2020]. In wider society, homeless people were housed in hotels [MINISTRY OF HOUSING 2020], and thousands of people put themselves forwards as NHS volunteers through the Royal Voluntary Service [NHS VOLUNTEER RESPONDERS 2021].

At the start of the crisis, staff adopted completely new ways of working almost overnight to ensure both patients and staff could be protected as much as possible from this unknown virus. NHS staff were labelled heroes and the UK vaccination programme was among the most efficient in the world [SHEPHEARD, M 2021]. However, as the crisis dragged on, the long-forgotten doorstep claps were replaced with increasing levels of criticism from some sections of the media, along with abuse from patients, angry and frustrated with the multiple knock-on effects this pandemic has created [BLAKEY, A WILKINSON, D 2021]. GPs bore the brunt of much of this anger, as many patients struggled to gain the access they were used to

Despite the efforts of the people of the NHS, they were working within a system that was already broken by years of austerity before the pandemic arrived and it can be safely said, that the response of the UK leadership was not 'world beating' when it came to coping with Covid-19. As of October 2021, the UK had the highest number of deaths from coronavirus in Western Europe (136,986 deaths or 2,029 deaths per million people), with over 7 million confirmed cases [STATISTA 2021]. The economy was recovering from a recession, while unemployment and national debt soared [SHEPHEARD, M 2021].

Tracing the timeline of events of the pandemic response in the UK tells the story of how this crisis unfolded. When other countries closed borders and locked down, the UK dallied and debated herd immunity. Contact tracing was abandoned in early March 2020 [PHE 2020b], while large gatherings continued to take place up until the end of that same month [CALVERT 2020].

Meanwhile, the faces on the frontlines, NHS and social care staff were left woefully unprotected by a lack of personal protective equipment (PPE). In 2016, a pandemic simulation exercise (Exercise Cygnus) had been carried out to demonstrate the effects of an influenza pandemic on the UK. It showed that the UK was not ready to cope with a pandemic, revealing a shortage of critical care beds, ventilators and PPE. The then Health secretary Jeremy Hunt reportedly voted against stockpiling gowns and visors due to the expense [CALVERT 2020].

Staff raised concerns at the outset of the pandemic, reporting the shortages were putting them at risk. The government confirmed in June 2020 that they had sourced and supplied a further 2 billion items of PPE to staff in England (numbers boosted by counting individual gloves rather than pairs [DIXON H 2020]). However, a BMA survey found that half of doctors working in high risk areas reported shortages of gowns and goggles [COOPER, K 2020], while many care homes reported paying inflated prices to source their own supplies [SAVAGE, M 2020].

The importance of this protection was highlighted in a BMJ study from China, which showed that healthcare workers who were appropriately attired with PPE did not contract Covid-19 while working in highly exposed environments [LIU, M et al 2020]. By early May 2020, twenty-nine healthcare workers had died from covid-19 in China. In the UK, 163 healthcare workers had died in the same time period. General practitioners were the highest risk specialty for deaths among doctors, while the highest risk nursing specialty was mental health [Bandyopadhyay S et al 2020]. There have been disproportionately high death rates among NHS staff from minority-ethnic backgrounds [COOK, T 2020].

Questions still need to be answered for the families of the thousands of people who have died during the pandemic – whether due to coronavirus itself, or due to the knock-on effects of the crisis. An inquiry into the government's handling of the pandemic has been promised by Boris Johnson, but is yet to be delivered. Major government decisions need to be investigated to ensure that when future pandemics strike – the same mistakes are avoided. The events of March 2020 were sadly repeated in December 2020 in an effort to 'save Christmas' [MCKEE, M 2021]. Decisions on the timing of lockdowns; plans to reopen schools; the cancelling of all elective surgeries; Nightingale hospitals that were barely used; the lack of initial testing for healthcare workers; the return of elderly patients from hospitals to care homes, and on major public procurement programmes such as those for PPE and on test and trace [SHEPHEARD, M 2021].

It is essential to have a health system that functions during times of crisis and this pandemic has highlighted both the gaping cracks in our NHS, and the huge health inequalities between different communities. It is convenient for those leading the country to line up scapegoats for the failures during the pandemic – to deflect the blame away from their own shortcomings. GPs have been in the firing line, Public Health England was axed, and even patients have been blamed for not following the ever-changing government advice. Attributing blame is a divisive distraction, and moving forward, conversations are needed on the sort of health service we want for this country.

If millions can be siphoned into untried ventures such as test and trace, then those in power can make choices to spend money on the areas of need within our health system. Areas such as staff welfare – ensuring the bare basics are covered so staff can eat, drink and take a break on shift – which sounds obvious but is so often lacking for staff working long shifts within the NHS, and rested staff provide a better service for patients. Go one step further and make the workplace appealing so staff stick around and workloads can be shared – enable flexible working, embrace telemedicine and tap into a whole new workforce such as those with caring responsibilities or those based overseas. Educate children from an early age on what the NHS is and what it is not – teach them how to use it and invest in health promotion. Address bureaucracy and invest in digital technology so that all NHS providers have access to the same systems [WELCH, E 2021, HODES, S et al 2021].

Few lives have been left untouched by the impact of this pandemic, and it has demonstrated how our world can be transformed during times of need – for better as well as for worse. There have, of course, been many positive outcomes too.

The use of technology within the NHS has leapt forward. A service still using fax machines, transitioned very quickly to using remote technology to enable clinicians throughout the service to consult remotely to keep patients safe. Home working is now imminently more possible with its myriad benefits for a jaded workforce. For housebound patients, or those living miles from health services, the use of such technology has transformed their experience. Similarly for patients seeking therapy for mental health problems – a virtual session may be more accessible.

On a larger level, the pandemic caused a major drop in pollution when the worldwide lockdowns were in force, brought on by a dramatic fall in travel, which in itself saved lives. During two weeks of lockdown, the number of cases of asthma in children reduced by 6,600 across twenty-seven countries – reminding us of the often overlooked health consequences of normal life [BURKE, M 2020].

It also demonstrated the power of the everyday person to make a difference. We watched a 99 year old man become a household name as

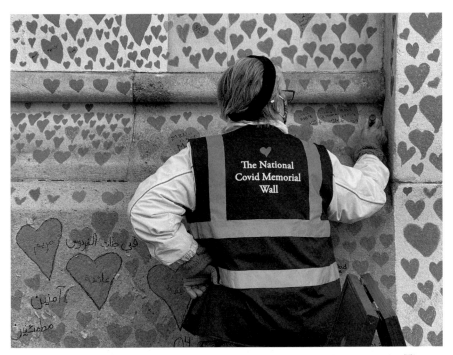

The National Covid Memorial Wall – 150,000 hearts stretch 500m along the Thames opposite Parliament. Each heart, drawn by volunteers, represents someone loved who lost their lives to Covid (*John Cameron on Unsplash*)

he attempted to raise money for NHS workers doing laps of his garden. Captain Sir Tom Moore amassed millions more than his £1,000 target, striking a cord with the public. We saw thousands of people volunteer to help deliver shopping and medicines to the housebound, and we realised the value of the keyworkers who kept the country functioning.

For the thousands of people who have died during this crisis, and their loved ones, it is important that lessons are learned, so that when the next pandemic comes our way – we have a health service that is fortified and united and able to cope.

References

ADEBOWALE, V ET AL (2020) Covid-19: Call for a rapid forward looking review of the uk's preparedness for a second wave – an open letter to the leaders of all UK political parties. BMJ https://www.bmj.com/content/369/bmj.m2514

AFP (2020) Hong Kong unveils virus quarantine plans, with jail for dodgers. https://hongkongfp.com/2020/02/07/hong-kong-unveils-virus-quarantine-plans-jail-dodgers/

AL-MUGHARABI, N., (2020). 'Gaza's health system days from being overwhelmed by COVID-19, advisers say' Reuters 25th November 2020. Accessed 4th February 2021. https://www.reuters.com/article/health-coronavirus-palestinians-gaza-int-idUSKBN2842WR

ALDI (2021) Aldi Graduate Area Manager Programme. https://www.aldirecruitment.co.uk/area-manager-programme/graduate-area-manager-programme

ANDERSON KG, RAMBAUT, A, LIPKIN WI, HOLMES EC, GARRY, RF (2020) The proximal origin of SARS-CoV-2. Nature Medicine 26, 450-452 https://www.nature.com/articles/s41591-020-0820-9

ANTONELLI, M, CAPDEVILA, J, CHAUDHARI, A., ET AL (2021) Optimal symptom combinations to aid COVID-19 case identification: Analysis from a community-based, prospective, observational cohort. Journal of infection 82, 3: 384-390 https://www.journalofinfection.com/article/S0163-4453(21)00079-7/fulltext#%20

ASSOCIATED PRESS (2020) Singapore covid-19 cases reach record, surge past 8,000. The Diplomat. 21 April 2020. https://thediplomat.com/2020/04/singapore-covid-19-cases-reach-record-surge-past-8000/

AUSTRALIAN GOVERNMENT DEPARTMENT OF HEALTH (AGDH 2020) What you need to know about Covid-19 https://www.health.gov.au/news/health-alerts/novel-coronavirus-2019-ncov-health-alert/what-you-need-to-know-about-coronavirus-covid-19

AVERT (2020) History of HIV and AIDS. https://www.avert.org/professionals/history-hiv-aids/overview

Bandyopadhyay S, Baticulon RE, Kadhum M, et al (2020) Infection and mortality of healthcare workers worldwide from COVID-19: a systematic review BMJ Global Health 5:e003097 https://gh.bmj.com/content/5/12/e003097#DC9

BBC (31 Jan 2020a) Coronavirus: Two cases confirmed in UK https://www.bbc.co.uk/news/health-51325192

BBC (1 May 2020b) Coronavirus: Trump stands by China lab origin theory for virus https://www.bbc.co.uk/news/world-us-canada-52496098

BBC (15 March 2020c) Coronavirus: Supermarkets ask shoppers to be considerate and stop stockpiling https://www.bbc.co.uk/news/business-51883440

BBC (1 April 2020d) Coronavirus: Boris Johnson vows more virus tests as UK deaths exceed 2,000 https://www.bbc.co.uk/news/uk-52122761

BBC (12 April 2020e) Coronavirus: 'Sombre day' as UK deaths hit 10,000. https://www.bbc.co.uk/news/uk-52264145

BBC (15 April 2020f) Coronavirus: Trump's WHO de-funding 'as dangerous as it sounds' https://www.bbc.co.uk/news/world-us-canada-52291654

BBC (2 May 2020g) Coronavirus: Government pledges £76m for abuse victims https://www.bbc.co.uk/news/uk-52516433

BBC (19 May 2020h) Coronavirus:Care homes should have been prioritized from the start MPs told https://www.bbc.co.uk/news/uk-52727221

BBC (10 June 2020i) Coronavirus: 'Earlier lockdown would have halved death toll' https://www.bbc.co.uk/news/health-52995064

BBC (25 June 2020j) Bournemouth beach: 'Major incident' as thousands flock to coast https://www.bbc.co.uk/news/uk-england-dorset-53176717

BBC (3 July 2020k) Leicester lockdown: New laws come into force https://www.bbc.co.uk/news/uk-england-leicestershire-53283967

BBC (17 July 2020l) Capt Sir Tom Moore knighted in 'unique' ceremony. https://www.bbc.co.uk/news/uk-england-beds-bucks-herts-53442746

BBC (5 August 2020m) Coronavirus: UK made serious mistake over border policy, say MPs https://www.bbc.co.uk/news/uk-politics-53654644

BBC (2 October 2020n) Covid-19: Boris Johnson says everybody got 'complacent' https://www.bbc.co.uk/news/uk-54392187

BBC (13 October 2020o) Covid: Sage scientists called for short lockdown weeks ago https://www.bbc.co.uk/news/uk-54518002

BBC (12 August 2021a) NHS waiting list in England hits record 5.45 million. https://www.bbc.co.uk/news/health-58186708

BBC (12 January 2021b) Covid-19: Care home boss moves back in with residents over outbreak fear. https://www.bbc.co.uk/news/uk-england-somerset-55626068

BERGER, D., (2021) Up the line to death: covid-19 has revealed a mortal betrayal of the world's healthcare workers. BMJ Blogs. January 29 2021. https://blogs.bmj.com/bmj/2021/01/29/up-the-line-to-death-covid-19-has-revealed-a-mortal-betrayal-of-the-worlds-healthcare-workers/

BHAGAWATI, D., (2021) NHS workers lost to covid 'deserve more'. Politics.co.uk. 25 March 2021. https://www.politics.co.uk/comment/2021/03/25/nhs-workers-lost-to-covid-deserve-more/

BLACKALL, M., (2020) UK care home covid-19 deaths 'may be five times government estimate' The Guardian. 18 April 2020. https://www.theguardian.com/world/2020/apr/18/uk-care-home-covid-19-deaths-may-be-five-times-government-estimate

BLAKEY, A,. WILKINSON, D,. (2021) 'Appalling' attack on GP surgery staff condemned after four injured in 'life-threatening' disturbance. Manchester Evening News. 18 Sep 2021.https://www.manchestereveningnews.co.uk/news/greater-manchester-news/appalling-attack-gp-surgery-staff-21607333

BMA (2020) The hidden impact of COVID-19 on patient care in the NHS in England. July 2020 https://www.bma.org.uk/media/2840/the-hidden-impact-of-covid_web-pdf.pdf

BMJ BEST PRACTICE (2021) Patient information from BMJ COVID-19 01 June 2021 https://bestpractice.bmj.com/patient-leaflets/en-us/pdf/3000166/Coronavirus.pdf

BMJ (2021) Remembering the UK doctors who have died of covid-19. https://www.bmj.com/covid-memorial

BOSELEY, S., (2020) WHO warns that few have developed antibodies to Covid-19. The Guardian. 20 April 2020. https://www.theguardian.com/society/2020/apr/20/studies-suggest-very-few-have-had-covid-19-without-symptoms

BOSELEY, S., ELGOT, J (2020) Liverpool to pioneer UK's first attempt at mass covid testing. The Guardian. 2 Nov 2020. https://www.theguardian.com/uk-news/2020/nov/02/liverpool-uk-first-attempt-coronavirus-mass-testing

BRIGGS A., JENKINS D, FRASER C. (2020) NHS Test and Trace: the journey so far. The Health Foundation. https://www.health.org.uk/sites/default/files/2020-09/NHS%20Test%20and%20Trace.pdf]

British Foreign Policy Group (BFPG 2020). COVID-19 Timeline. https://bfpg.co.uk/2020/04/covid-19-timeline/

BRYNER J., (2020) 1st known case of coronavirus traced back to November in China. Live Science. March 14 2020 https://www.livescience.com/first-case-coronavirus-found.html

BUCHAN, L., (2020) Government to write off £13.4bn in historic NHS debt amid coronavirus crisis. Independent. 2 April 2020 https://www.independent.co.uk/news/uk/politics/coronavirus-nhs-debt-matt-hancock-press-conference-briefing-a9443926.html

CALISHER C., Carroll D, COLWELL, R, CORLEY RB, DASZAK P, DROSTEN C et al (2020) Statement in support of the scientists, public health professionals and medical professionals of China combatting COVID-19. The Lancet. 395, 10226, E42-43 https://www.thelancet.com/journals/lancet/article/PIIS0140-6736(20)30418-9/fulltext

CALVERT, J., ARBUTHNOTT, G., LEAKE, J. (2020) Coronavirus: 38 days when Britain sleepwalked into disaster. The Sunday Times. April 19 2020. https://www.thetimes.co.uk/article/coronavirus-38-days-when-britain-sleepwalked-into-disaster-hq3b9tlgh

CAMPBELL, D., (2019) Why is Matt Hancock bringing bursaries back for student nurses? The Guardian 18 December 2019 https://www.theguardian.com/society/2019/dec/18/why-is-matt-hancock-bringing-bursaries-back-for-student-nurses

CAMPBELL, D., (2020) Growing numbers of NHS nurses quit within three years study finds. The Guardian. 23 September 2020 https://www.theguardian.com/society/2020/sep/23/growing-numbers-of-nhs-nurses-quit-within-three-years-study-finds

CARMICHAEL, C., (2021) What's the typical starting wage for a Nurse in the UK in 2021. https://www.nurses.co.uk/nursing/blog/what-s-the-typical-starting-wage-for-a-nurse-in-the-uk-in-2021/

CARRINGTON, D., (2020) UK road travel falls to 1955 levels as covid-19 lockdown takes hold. The Guardian. 3 April 2020. https://www.theguardian.com/uk-news/2020/apr/03/uk-road-travel-falls-to-1955-levels-as-covid-19-lockdown-takes-hold-coronavirus-traffic

Centre for Evidence-Based Medicine (2020) Covid-19: Admissions to Hospital update. 1 May 2020. https://www.cebm.net/covid-19/covid-19-uk-hospital-admissions/

CHARLES, A, EWBANK, L, McKENNA, H, WENZEL, L., (2019) The NHS long-term plan explained. The King's Fund https://www.kingsfund.org.uk/publications/nhs-long-term-plan-explained

CHOI, Y.J., (2020) COVID-19 in South Korea. Postgrad Med. J; 96: 399-402 https://pmj.bmj.com/content/postgradmedj/96/1137/399.full.pdf

The Centre for Health Protection (CHP 2020). CHP closely monitors clusters of pneumonia on mainland. https://www.info.gov.hk/gia/general/201912/31/P2019123100667.htm

COGORA (2021) Press Release: Pulse most widely read non-reference journal among GPs. 10 August 2021. https://www.cogora.com/pulse-most-widely-read-non-reference-journal-among-gps/

COHEN, E., SAYERS, DM. (2020) 108 potential Covid-19 vaccines in the works worldwide. CNN. 5 May 2020 https://edition.cnn.com/world/live-news/coronavirus-pandemic-05-05-20-intl/h_ffcb19f55361a521544afb1bf66ddde5

COOK, T., KURSUMOVIC, E., LENNANE, S. (2020) Exclusive: deaths of NHS staff from covid-19 analysed. HSJ https://www.hsj.co.uk/exclusive-deaths-of-nhs-staff-from-covid-19-analysed/7027471.article

COOPER, J., (2018) Jews in the National Health Service: from refugees to medicine's cutting edge. The J C https://www.thejc.com/news/uk/jews-in-the-nhs-from-refugees-to-medicine-s-cutting-edge-1.474347

COOPER, K., (2020) BAME doctors hit worse by lack of PPE. BMA. https://www.bma.org.uk/news-and-opinion/bame-doctors-hit-worse-by-lack-of-ppe

DAUK (2020) Doctors win a reimbursement for the Immigration Health Surcharge. https://www.dauk.org/news/2020/06/10/immigrationhealthsurcharge kickintheteet/

DAYAN, M., (2020) Chart of the week: NHS staff pay and the cost of living. Nuffield Trust. https://www.nuffieldtrust.org.uk/resource/chart-of-the-week-nhs-staff-pay-and-the-cost-of-living

DEPARTMENT FOR BUSINESS (2020) Call for businesses to help make NHS ventilators. 16 March 2020 https://www.gov.uk/government/news/production-and-supply-of-ventilators-and-ventilator-components

Department of Health and Social Care (2020a) Press release. COVID-19: government announces moving out of contain phase and into delay. https://www.gov.uk/government/news/covid-19-government-announces-moving-out-of-contain-phase-and-into-delay

Department of Health and Social Care (2020b) Guidance on care home visiting https://www.gov.uk/government/publications/visiting-care-homes-during-coronavirus/update-on-policies-for-visiting-arrangements-in-care-homes

Department of Health and Social Care (2020c) Government creates new National Institute for Health Protection. 18 August 2020 https://www.gov.uk/government/news/government-creates-new-national-institute-for-health-protection

DHSC (2020) 29 February 2020. Available at: https://twitter.com/dhscgovuk/status/1233754536856125441?lang=en

DISCOMBE, M., (2020) Medical students and new doctors could be drafted in to fight coronavirus. Health Service Journal. March 5 2020 https://www.hsj.co.uk/acute-care/medical-students-and-new-doctors-could-be-drafted-in-to-fight-coronavirus/7027060.article

DIXON, H., (2020) PPE: Government counter each glove as single item to reach one billion total investigation shows. 28 April 2020. https://www.telegraph.co.uk/politics/2020/04/28/ppe-government-counted-glove-single-item-reach-one-billion-total/

DUNCAN, C., (2020) Coronavirus: How Boris Johnson ignored health advice at his peril before Covid-19 diagnosis. Independent.27 March 2020. https://www.independent.co.uk/news/uk/politics/coronavirus-boris-johnson-positive-test-health-advice-shaking-hands-hospital-hancock-a9430231.html

DUNHILL, L., (2020) Critical care unit overwhelmed by coronavirus patients. HSJ. 20 March 2020 https://www.hsj.co.uk/news/exclusive-critical-care-unit-overwhelmed-by-coronavirus-patients/7027189.article

ECONOMIST (2020) Italy faces a sudden surge in covid-19 cases. 23 Feb 2020. https://www.economist.com/europe/2020/02/23/italy-faces-a-sudden-surge-in-covid-19-cases

ELLIOTT, L., STEWART, H. (2020) Budget 2020: Rishi Sunak turns on taps with £30bn splurge. The Guardian. 11 March 2020. https://www.theguardian.com/uk-news/2020/mar/11/budget-2020-rishi-sunak-spending-coronavirus

ESMAIL A., (2007) Asian doctors in the NHS:service and betrayal. British Journal of General Practice; 57 (543):827-834

EWBANK, L., THOMPSON, J, McKENNA, H, ANANDACIVA, S,. (2020) NHS hospital bed numbers. The King's Fund https://www.kingsfund.org.uk/publications/nhs-hospital-bed-numbers

GALLAGHER, P., (2020) Coronavirus latest: Sir Patrick Vallance admits UK failed to ramp up testing quickly enough. inews. 5 May 2020 https://

inews.co.uk/news/coronavirus-sir-patrick-vallance-admits-uk-failed-testing-capacity-424986

GALLAGHER, J., (2020) Coronavirus: Key evidence on opening schools revealed. 22 May 2020 https://www.bbc.co.uk/news/health-52770355

GEDDES, L., (2020) Four-week cancer treatment delay raises death risk by 10%-study. The Guardian. 4 November 2020 https://www.theguardian.com/society/2020/nov/04/four-week-cancer-treatment-delay-raises-death-risk-study-nhs-covid

GHOSH, P., (2020) Coronavirus: Some scientists say UK virus strategy is risking lives. BBC. 15 March 2020 https://www.bbc.co.uk/news/science-environment-51892402

GMC (2019) Fair to Refer? Reducing disproportionality in fitness to practise concerns reported to the GMC. https://www.gmc-uk.org/-/media/documents/fair-to-refer-report_pdf-79011677.pdf

GMC (2020) Covid-19: GMC grants temporary registration to 11,800 doctors. 27 March 2020. https://www.gmc-uk.org/news/news-archive/coronavirus---gmc-grants-temporary-registration-to-11800-doctors

GONG, S., BAO, L (2018) The battle against SARS and MERS coronaviruses: Reservoirs and animal models. Animal Mod Exp Med 1 (2): 125-133 https://www.ncbi.nlm.nih.gov/pmc/articles/PMC6388065/

GOV.UK (2020a) Press release: PM announces new funding in fight against spread of coronavirus. 6 March 2020 https://www.gov.uk/government/news/pm-announces-new-funding-in-fight-against-spread-of-coronavirus

GOV.UK (2020b) Press release: New government partnership with airlines to fly back more tourists stranded abroad. 30 March 2020. https://www.gov.uk/government/news/new-government-partnership-with-airlines-to-fly-back-more-tourists-stranded-abroad

GOV.UK (2021) UK Coronavirus dashboard. https://coronavirus.data.gov.uk/details/cases?_ga=2.251924238.642576993.1633560334-1144244331.1611791311

GREEN, A., (2020) Li Wenliang. The Lancet, 395, 10225: 682 https://www.thelancet.com/journals/lancet/article/PIIS0140-6736(20)30382-2/fulltext

HAMMOUDEH, W, KIENZLER, H, MEAGHER K., et al (2020) Social and political determinants of health in the occupied Palestine territory (oPt) during the COVID-19 pandemic: who is responsible? *BMJ Global Health* 2020;5:e003683 https://gh.bmj.com/content/bmjgh/5/9/e003683.full.pdf

HARDING, L., (2020a) 'Weird as hell': the covid-19 patients who have symptoms for months. The Guardian. May 15 2020 https://www.theguardian.com/world/2020/may/15/weird-hell-professor-advent-calendar-covid-19-symptoms-paul-garner

HARDING, L., (2020b) 'It feels endless': Four women struggling to recover from Covid-19. The Guardian. June 7 2020 https://www.theguardian.com/world/2020/jun/07/it-feels-endless-four-women-struggling-to-recover-from-covid-19-coronavirus-symptoms

HASAN, R., (2020) BAME medical groups write to health secretary demanding urgent action to safeguard them from further coronavirus deaths. ITV 7 June 2020 https://www.itv.com/news/2020-06-07/bame-medical-groups-write-to-health-secretary-demanding-urgent-action-to-safeguard-them-from-further-coronavirus-deaths

HIGGETT K., et al (2020) NHS to free up 30,000 beds for coronavirus. HSJ 17 March 2020. https://www.hsj.co.uk/free-for-non-subscribers/nhs-to-free-up-30000-beds-for-coronavirus/7027148.article

HILL, E., TIEFENTHALER, A, TRIEBERT, C, JORDAN, D, WILLIS, H, STEIN, R. (2020) How George Floyd was killed in Police Custody. New York Times. (updated 20 April 2021) https://www.nytimes.com/2020/05/31/us/george-floyd-investigation.html

HOLMES, E., (2020). Initial genome release of novel coronavirus 2020 [14 January 2020]. Available from: http://virological.org/t/initial-genome-release-of-novel-coronavirus/319

HM Revenue and Customs (2020) Get a discount with the Eat Out to Help Our scheme. https://www.gov.uk/guidance/get-a-discount-with-the-eat-out-to-help-out-scheme

HODES, S., HUSSAIN,S., JHA, N., TOBERTY,L., WELCH,E. (2021) If general practice fails, the NHS fails. BMJ Blogs May 14 2021 https://blogs.bmj.com/bmj/2021/05/14/if-general-practice-fails-the-nhs-fails/

HOLSHUE, M.L., ET AL (2020) First Case of 2019 Novel Coronavirus in the United States. N Engl J Med, 382: 929-936 https://www.nejm.org/doi/full/10.1056/NEJMoa2001191

HOWIE, M. (2021) Britain's Covid infection rate is one of the worst in the world, data reveals. Evening Standard.2 October 2021. https://www.standard.co.uk/news/uk/uk-covid-infection-rate-global-comparison-johns-hopkins-who-b958154.html

HUANG, C et al, (2020) Clinical features of patients infected with 2019 novel coronavirus in Wuhan, China. *The Lancet*, 395, 10223: 497-506 https://www.thelancet.com/journals/lancet/article/PIIS0140-6736(20)30183-5/fulltext

IBRAHIM, A., (2020) Two die of coronavirus in Iran, first fatalities in the Middle East. Al Jazeera 19 Feb 2020 https://www.aljazeera.com/news/2020/2/19/two-die-of-coronavirus-in-iran-first-fatalities-in-middle-east

ILLMAN, J., (2020) NHS block books almost all private hospital sector capacity to fight covid-19. HSJ. 21 March 2020 https://www.hsj.co.uk/policy-and-regulation/nhs-block-books-almost-all-private-hospital-sector-capacity-to-fight-covid-19/7027196.article

IMAI, N. et al (2020) Report 3. Transmissibility of 2019-nCoV. Imperial College London COVID-19 Response Team. https://www.imperial.ac.uk/media/imperial-college/medicine/sph/ide/gida-fellowships/Imperial-College-COVID19-transmissibility-25-01-2020.pdf

JOHN HOPKINS UNIVERSITY (2021) Coronavirus Resource Centre. https://coronavirus.jhu.edu/map.html

JONES, A., (2020) How did New Zealand become Covid-19 free? BBC News. 10 July 2020. https://www.bbc.co.uk/news/world-asia-53274085

KAFFASH, J. PHILPOTTS, E., (2020) Exclusive: Covid vaccine DES set to be announced imminently for December start. https://www.pulsetoday.co.uk/news/breaking-news/covid-vaccine-des-set-to-be-announced-imminently-for-december-start/

KASPRZAK, E., (2019) Why are black mothers at more risk of dying? BBC News https://www.bbc.co.uk/news/uk-england-47115305\

KEANE, M., NEAL, T., (2020) Consumer panic in the COVID-19 pandemic. Journal of Econometrics https://www.sciencedirect.com/science/article/pii/S0304407620302840?via%3Dihub

KELION, L., (2020) Coronavirus: 20 suspected phone mast attacks over Easter. BBC 14 April 2020. https://www.bbc.co.uk/news/technology-52281315

KEOGH, K., JONES-BERRY, S, KENDALL-RAYNOR, P, HACKETT, K (2021) COVID-19: remembering the nursing staff who have lost their lives. Nursing Standard. 17 February 2021 https://rcni.com/nursing-standard/features/covid-19-remembering-nursing-staff-who-have-lost-their-lives-160011

KNAPTON, S., BODKIN, H (2020) PHE warned in February against discharges into care homes where there was risk of coronavirus transmission. 5 June 2020. The Telegraph https://www.telegraph.co.uk/politics/2020/06/05/phe-warned-february-against-discharges-care-homes-risk-coronavirus/

KNIGHT, M, BUNCH, K, TUFFNELL, D, JAYAKODY, H, SHAKESPEARE, J, KOTNIS, R, KENYON, S, KURINCZUK, J.J., (2018) Saving Lives, Improving Mothers' Care Lessons lerned to inform maternity care from the UK and Ireland Confidential Enquiries into Maternal Deaths and Morbidity 2014-16. https://www.npeu.ox.ac.uk/downloads/files/mbrrace-uk/reports/MBRRACE-UK%20Maternal%20Report%202018%20-%20Web%20Version.pdf

KOH, D., (2020) Singapore government launches new app for contact tracing to combat spread of covid-19. Mobi Health News. 20 March 2020. https://www.mobihealthnews.com/news/apac/singapore-government-launches-new-app-contact-tracing-combat-spread-covid-19

The Lancet Infectious Diseases (2020). The COVID-19 infodemic. Lancet Infect Dis. 2020 Aug;20(8):875. doi: 10.1016/S1473-3099(20)30565-X. https://www.thelancet.com/journals/laninf/article/PIIS1473-3099(20)30565-X/fulltext

LESTER JC, JIA JL, ZHANG L, OKOYE GA, LINOS E., (2020) Absence of images of skin of colour in publications of COVID-19 skin manifestations. British Journal of Dermatology https://doi.org/10.1111/bjd.19258

LI, S., (2020) As Coronavirus spreads, so does anti-Chinese racism. Teen Vogue https://www.teenvogue.com/story/coronavirus-anti-chinese-racism

LINTON, S., (2020) Taking the difference out of attainment. BMJ; 368 https://www.bmj.com/content/368/bmj.m438

LINTERN, S., (2020b) NHS workforce 'could not cope' with third wave. The Independent. 30 November 2020 https://www.independent.co.uk/news/health/coronavirus-nhs-hospitals-staff-nurses-doctors-b1764074.html

LINTERN, S., (2021) Almost 200,000 patients now waiting at least a year for routine NHS operation. The Independent 14 January 2021 https://www.independent.co.uk/news/health/nhs-waiting-times-operations-b1787154.html

LIU, M, et al (2020) Use of personal protective equipment against coronavirus disease 2019 by healthcare professionals in Wuhan, China: cross sectional study. BMJ 2020; 369: https://doi.org/10.1136/bmj.m2195

LOVETT, S., (2020) Teachers' unions condemn 'reckless' school plans as 390,000 sign petition demanding parents given choice to keep children at home. Independent. 11 May 2020. https://www.independent.co.uk/news/uk/home-news/coronavirus-schools-uk-covid-19-latest-return-date-june-exams-children-a9508456.html

MAHASE, E., (2020) Vaccinating the UK: how the covid vaccine was approved and other questions answered. BMJ 2020; 371: m 4759 https://www.bmj.com/content/371/bmj.m4759

MAJID, A., (2020) What lies beneath: getting under the skin of GMC referrals. BMJ; 368 https://www.bmj.com/content/368/bmj.m338

MCCONKEY, R. WYATT, S., (2020) Exploring the fall in A&E visits during the pandemic. The Health Foundation. https://www.health.org.uk/news-and-comment/charts-and-infographics/exploring-the-fall-in-a-e-visits-during-the-pandemic

MCCURRY J, RATCLIFFE R, DAVIDSON D (2020) Mass testing, alerts and big fines: the strategies used in Asia to slow coronavirus. https://www.theguardian.com/world/2020/mar/11/mass-testing-alerts-and-big-fines-the-strategies-used-in-asia-to-slow-coronavirus]

MCFARLING, U.L., (2020) Dermatology faces a reckoning: Lack of darker skin in textbooks and journals harms care for patients of color. Statnews https://www.statnews.com/2020/07/21/dermatology-faces-reckoning-lack-of-darker-skin-in-textbooks-journals-harms-patients-of-color/

MCINTYRE, N., DUNCAN, P. (2020) Care homes and coronavirus: why we don't know the true UK death toll. The Guardian. 14 April 2020. https://www.theguardian.com/world/2020/apr/14/care-homes-coronavirus-why-we-dont-know-true-uk-death-toll

MCKEE, M., (2021) What went wrong in the UK's covid-19 response.. BMJ 373:n1309 https://www.bmj.com/content/373/bmj.n1309

MCLAUGHLIN A., (2020) Investigating the most convincing covid-19 conspiracy theories. 23 June 2020. https://www.kcl.ac.uk/investigating-the-most-convincing-covid-19-conspiracy-theories

MINISTRY OF HOUSING (2020) £3.2 million emergency support for rough sleepers during coronavirus outbreak. 17 March 2020. https://www.gov.uk/government/news/3-2-million-emergency-support-for-rough-sleepers-during-coronavirus-outbreak

MORAN-THOMAS, A., (2020) How a popular medical device encodes racial bias. Boston Review http://bostonreview.net/science-nature-race/amy-moran-thomas-how-popular-medical-devices. -encodes-racial-bias

MORIARTY, L.F., et al (2020) Public Health Responses to COVID-19 Outbreaks on Cruise Ships – Worldwide, February-March 2020. CDC, 69 (12); 347-352 https://www.cdc.gov/mmwr/volumes/69/wr/mm6912e3.htm

NHS CHARITIES TOGETHER (2021) Our tribute to Captain Sir Tom Moore. Feb 2 2021. https://www.nhscharitiestogether.co.uk/our-tribute-to-captain-sir-tom-moore/

NHS CONFEDERATION (2020) The impact of covid-19 on BME communities and health and care staff. Member briefing April 2020 https://www.nhsconfed.org/-/media/Confederation/Files/Publications/Documents/BRIEFING_Impact-of-COVID-19-BME_communities-and-staff_FNL.pdf?dl=1

NHS DIGITAL (2019) NHS Workforce Statistics – March 2019. https://digital.nhs.uk/data-and-information/publications/statistical/nhs-workforce-statistics/nhs-workforce-statistics---march-2019-provisional-statistics

NHS DIGITAL (2020) NHS Workforce Statistics – June 2020. https://digital.nhs.uk/data-and-information/publications/statistical/nhs-workforce-statistics/june-2020

NHS DIGITAL (2021) Appointments in General Practice. 30 September 2021. https://digital.nhs.uk/data-and-information/publications/statistical/appointments-in-general-practice#latest-statistics

NHS ENGLAND (2019) NHS Workforce Race Equality Standard report. https://www.england.nhs.uk/wp-content/uploads/2020/01/wres-2019-data-report.pdf

NHS PROVIDERS (2020) Government updates. April 2020. https://nhsproviders.org/topics/covid-19/coronavirus-member-support/national-guidance/government-updates/daily-updates/april-2020

NHS VOLUNTEER RESPONDERS (2021) https://nhsvolunteerresponders.org.uk

NICE (2020) COVID-19 rapid guideline: managing the long-term effects of COVID-19. 18 December 2020 https://www.nice.org.uk/guidance/ng188

NMC (2020) NMC Covid-19 emergency register goes live with more than 7,000 former nurses and midwives ready to support health and social care services across the UK. 27 March 2020 https://www.nmc.org.uk/news/press-releases/nmc-covid-19-emergency-register-goes-live/

NPCC (2020) Policing the pandemic: The Health Protetion (Coronavirus restrictions, England) (Amendment)(No 2) changes – 13 May 2020 https://www.nfuonline.com/nfu-online/science-and-environment/access-issues/npcc-health-protection-regulations-amendments-england-130520/

NURSING NOTES (2021) Memorial of Health and Social Care Workers taken by COVID-19. https://nursingnotes.co.uk/covid-19-memorial/#

OFFICE FOR NATIONAL STATISTICS. (2020a) Coronavirus (COVID-19) related deaths by ethnic group, England and

Wales: 2 March 2020 to 10 April 2020. https://www.ons.gov.uk/peoplepopulationandcommunity/birthsdeathsandmarriages/deaths/articles/coronavirusrelateddeathsbyethnicgroupenglandandwales/2march2020to10april2020

OFFICE FOR NATIONAL STATISTICS (2020b) Analysis of death registrationsnotinvolvingcoronavirus,EnglandandWales:28December2019to 1May2020. https://www.ons.gov.uk/peoplepopulationandcommunity/birthsdeathsandmarriages/deaths/articles/analysisofdeathregistrationsnotinvolvingcoronaviruscovid19englandandwales28december2019to1may2020/technical annex

OFFICE FOR NATIONAL STATISTICS (ONS) (2021) Coronavirus related deaths by occupation, England and Wales, deaths registered between 9 march and 28 december 2020 https://www.ons.gov.uk/peoplepopulationandcommunity/healthandsocialcare/causesofdeath/bulletins/coronaviruscovid19relateddeathsbyoccupationenglandandwales/deathsregisteredbetween9marchand28december2020

OXFORD VACCINE GROUP (2020) Oxford covid-19 vaccine begins human trial stage. 24 April 2020 https://www.ovg.ox.ac.uk/news/oxford-covid-19-vaccine-begins-human-trial-stage

PARLIAMENT PUBLICATIONS (2020) Readying the NHS and social care for the COVID-19 peak. 29 July 2020 https://publications.parliament.uk/pa/cm5801/cmselect/cmpubacc/405/40502.htm

PARVEEN, N., (2020) Priti Patel says sorry if people feel there have been failings over PPE. The Guardian. 11 April 2020. https://www.theguardian.com/world/2020/apr/11/priti-patel-says-sorry-if-people-feel-there-have-been-failings-over-ppe

PAUL, K., (2021) Facebook bans misinformation about all vaccines after years of controversy. The Guardian. 8 Feb 2021. https://www.theguardian.com/technology/2021/feb/08/facebook-bans-vaccine-misinformation

PESTON, R., (2020) Robert Peston: Is Michael Gove right that there is a shortage of test kit ingredients? 31 March 2020 https://www.itv.com/news/2020-03-31/robert-peston-is-gove-right-that-there-is-a-shortage-of-test-kit-ingredients

PHE (2016) Exercise Cygnus report Tier one command post exercise Pandemic Influenza. 18 to 20 October 2016 https://assets.publishing.service.gov.uk/government/uploads/system/uploads/attachment_data/file/927770/exercise-cygnus-report.pdf

PHE (2020a) Guidance for social or community care and residential settings on COVID-19. 25 February 2020 (withdrawn 13 March 2020) https://www.gov.uk/government/publications/guidance-for-social-or-community-care-and-residential-settings-on-covid-19/guidance-for-social-or-community-care-and-residential-settings-on-covid-19

PHE (2020b)COVID-19: guidance for households with possible coronavirus infection. 12 March 2020 (multiple subsequent updates) https://www.gov.uk/government/publications/covid-19-stay-at-home-guidance#history

PHILPOTTS, E., (2021) Tributes to Dr Kailash Chand OBE. Pulse. 27 July 2021 https://www.pulsetoday.co.uk/views/kailash-chand/tributes-to-dr-kailash-chand-obe/

PIDD, H., STEWART, H., SYAL, R., (2020) Johnson makes U-turn on free school meals after Rashford campaign. The Guardian. 16 June 2020 https://www.theguardian.com/politics/2020/jun/16/boris-johnson-faces-tory-rebellion-over-marcus-rashfords-school-meals-call

PULSE (2020) GPs come together to share homemade PPE amid shortage. 2 April 2020. https://www.pulsetoday.co.uk/news/coronavirus/gps-come-together-to-share-homemade-ppe-amid-shortage/

PULSE (2020a) Covid-19 deaths will be counted if person had positive virus test in past month. 13 August 2020 https://www.pulsetoday.co.uk/news/coronavirus/covid-19-deaths-will-be-counted-if-person-had-positive-virus-test-in-past-month/

PULSE (2020b) Tributes Page – GPs who sadly died with Covid-19. 22 April 2020. https://www.pulsetoday.co.uk/special/practice-life/tributes-page-gps-who-sadly-died-with-covid-19/

PULSE (2021a) Pulse features assistant wins two awards at magazine editors event. 2 July 2021 https://www.pulsetoday.co.uk/news/uncategorised/pulse-features-assistant-wins-two-awards-at-magazine-editors-event

PULSE (2021b) The media's anti-GP agenda. 2 Feb 2021. https://www.pulsetoday.co.uk/analysis/cover-feature/the-medias-anti-gp-agenda/

PULSE (2021c) Working Life: Mentoring primary care workers in rural Nepal. 4 June 2021 https://www.pulsetoday.co.uk/working-life/working-life/working-life-mentoring-primary-care-workers-in-rural-nepal/

PULSE (2021d) Working Life: Healthcare in the extremes. 20 August 2021. https://www.pulsetoday.co.uk/working-life/working-life/working-life-healthcare-in-the-extremes/

PULSE (2021e) Working Life: Connecting remote Zambia. 07 September 2021. https://www.pulsetoday.co.uk/working-life/working-life/working-life-connecting-remote-zambia/

QIN, A., et al (2020). China reports first death from new virus. New York Times https://www.nytimes.com/2020/01/10/world/asia/china-virus-wuhan-death.html

READ, S., (2020) Covid spending: Watchdog finds MPs' contacts were given priority. The Guardian. 18 November 2020 https://www.bbc.co.uk/news/business-54978460

REID, C., (2020) UK Government boosts bicycling and walking with ambitious 2 billion post pandemic plan. Forbes. 7 May 2020. https://www.forbes.com/sites/carltonreid/2020/05/09/uk-government-boosts-bicycling-and-walking-with-ambitious-2-billion-post-pandemic-plan/

REUTERS (2020) British Airways, Iberia suspend direct flights to mainland China amid virus fears. https://uk.reuters.com/article/us-china-health-britain-ba/british-airways-iberia-suspend-direct-flights-to-mainland-china-amid-virus-fears-idUKKBN1ZS0OJ

REUTERS IN PARIS (2020) French hospital discovers Covid-19 case from December. The Guardian. 4 May 2020 https://www.theguardian.com/world/2020/may/04/french-hospital-discovers-covid-19-case-december-retested

RIMMER, A., (2020) Almost a third of UK doctors may be burnt out and stressed, study suggests. BMJ; 368:m323 https://www.bmj.com/content/368/bmj.m323

ROBERTS, M., (2020) Understanding the dangerous 'false economy' of public health cuts. The National Health Executive. 2 Dec 2020 https://www.nationalhealthexecutive.com/articles/understanding-dangerous-false-economy-public-health-cuts

ROYAL COLLEGE OF NURSING (2020) BAME nursing staff experiencing greater PPE shortages despite COVID-19 risk warnings. https://www.rcn.org.uk/news-and-events/news/uk-bame-nursing-staff-experiencing-greater-ppe-shortages-covid-19-280520

SAGE (2020) Potential impact of behavioural and social interventions on a covid-19 epidemic in the UK https://assets.publishing.service.gov.uk/government/uploads/system/uploads/attachment_data/file/882718/21-potential-impact-behavioural-social-interventions-04032020.pdf

SAVAGE, M., (2020) UK care homes scramble to buy their own PPE as national deliveries fail. 9 May 2020. https://www.theguardian.com/world/2020/may/09/uk-care-homes-scramble-to-buy-their-own-ppe-as-national-deliveries-fail

SHEPHEARD, M., NORRIS, E., (2021) The coronavirus inquiry. The case for an investigation of government actions during the Covid-19 pandemic. April 2021 https://www.instituteforgovernment.org.uk/sites/default/files/publications/coronavirus-inquiry.pdf

SHRAER, R., (2020) Coronavirus: ExCeL Centre planned as NHS field hospital. BBC. 24 March 2020. https://www.bbc.co.uk/news/health-52018477

SIDDIQUE, H., (2020) UK Covid death toll rises by 241 in highest daily increase for months. The Guardian 20 October 2020. https://www.theguardian.com/world/2020/oct/20/uk-covid-death-toll-rises-biggest-daily-increase-coronavirus

SKY NEWS (2020) Coronavirus: How the UKs 14 day travel quarantine will work. 8 June 2020. https://news.sky.com/story/coronavirus-how-the-uks-14-day-travel-quarantine-will-work-11992551

SKY NEWS (2021). Three quarters of under 50s in hospital with coronavirus are unvaccinated figures reveal. 15 September 2021. https://news.sky.com/story/covid-three-quarters-of-under-50s-in-hospital-with-coronavirus-are-unvaccinated-figures-reveal-12398321

SMITH, N., et al (2020) China locks down 14 cities as Wuhan coronavirus spreads. The Telegraph https://www.telegraph.co.uk/news/2020/01/24/china-locks-eight-cities-pledges-new-hospital-within-six-days/

SPEARE-Cole, R., (2020) Coronavirus fears fail to dampen London Chinese New Year 2020 celebrations. Evening Standard https://www.standard.co.uk/news/london/london-chinese-new-year-coronavirus-a4344996.html

SPENCER, K., (2020) Coronavirus: NHS Nightingale Hospital for COVID-19 patients opened by Prince Charles. 3 April 2020. https://news.sky.com/story/coronavirus-nhs-nightingale-hospital-opened-by-prince-charles-11967757

STATISTA (2021) Cumulative number of coronavirus deaths in the United Kingdom. 4 October 2021. https://www.statista.com/statistics/1109595/coronavirus-mortality-in-the-uk/

THOMAS, K., PASCOE, R. (2018) Being Resilient. Learning from community responses to gangs in Cape Town. The Global Initiative against Transnational organized crime. https://globalinitiative.net/wp-content/uploads/2019/01/TGIATOC-ManenburgWeb-FA.pdf

THORNTON J., (2020) Ethnic minority patients receive worse mental healthcare than White patients, review finds. BMJ; 368: 1058 https://www.bmj.com/content/368/bmj.m1058

TRIGGLE, N., (2020) Coronavirus: One in five deaths now linked to virus. 14 April 2020. https://www.bbc.co.uk/news/health-52278825

TRUMP, D., (2020). 16 March Available at: https://twitter.com/realDonaldTrump/status/1239685852093169664

TUCKER, M., GOLDBERG, A. (2020) Coronavirus: Sports events in March caused increased suffering and death. 26 May 2020 https://www.bbc.co.uk/news/uk-52797002

UNCTAD (2020) Report: Economic costs of the Israeli occupation for the Palestinian people: the Gaza Strip under closure and restrictions. November 2020 https://unctad.org/system/files/official-document/a75d310_en_1.pdf

UNITED NATIONS (2021) The question of Palestine. Covid-19 WHO situation report 63. 11 February 2021 https://www.un.org/unispal/document/coronavirus-disease-2019-covid-19-who-situation-report-63/

VAGNONI G., (2020) Coronavirus came to Italy almost 6 months before the first official case, new study shows. World Economic Forum https://www.weforum.org/agenda/2020/11/coronavirus-italy-covid-19-pandemic-europe-date-antibodies-study

VAN ASTEN, L., HARMEN, C.N., STOELDRAIJER, L., et al (2021) Excess Deaths during Influenza and Coronavirus Disease and Infection-Fatality Rate for Severe Acute Respiratory Syndrome Coronavirus 2, the Netherlands. Emerg Infect Dis. 2021 Feb;27(2):411-420. doi: 10.3201/eid2702.202999. Epub 2021 Jan 4. PMID: 33395381. https://pubmed.ncbi.nlm.nih.gov/33395381/

WANG, C., et al (2020). A novel coronavirus outbreak of global health concern. The Lancet, 395, 10223: 470-473 https://www.thelancet.com/journals/lancet/article/PIIS0140-6736(20)30185-9/fulltext

WELCH, E., (2021) MPs may not have solutions for the burnout emergency among NHS staff, but doctors do. Independent. 12 June 2021 https://www.independent.co.uk/voices/nhs-burnout-pandemic-covid-b1864641.html

WENGER, M., (2016) Manenberg in dire need of more police. Ground up. 7 July 2016 https://www.groundup.org.za/article/manenberg-dire-need-more-police/

WFP (2020) Covid-19 will double number of people facing food crises unless swift action is taken. 21 April 2020. https://www.wfp.org/news/covid-19-will-double-number-people-facing-food-crises-unless-swift-action-taken

WHO (2003). Consensus document on the epidemiology of severe acute respiratory syndrome (SARS) https://www.who.int/csr/sars/en/WHOconsensus.pdf?ua=1

WHO (2015). WHO Best Practices for the naming of new human infectious diseases (Geneva: World Health Organisation, May 2015) https://apps.who.int/iris/bitstream/handle/10665/163636/WHO_HSE_FOS_15.1_eng.pdf;jsessionid=E693B4FE32A5F6593C46BCF0FFEEDFCC?sequence=1]

WHO (12 Jan 2020). Novel coronavirus – China. http://www.who.int/csr/don/12-january-2020-novel-coronavirus-china/en/

WHO (22 Jan 2020). Mission summary: WHO field visit to Wuhan, China 20-21 January 2020. https://www.who.int/china/news/detail/22-01-2020-field-visit-wuhan-china-jan-2020

WHO (2020a). Novel Coronavirus (2019-nCoV) SITUATION REPORTS. Weekly Epidemiologival Update and Weekly Operational Update Jan-Dec 2020 available at: https://www.who.int/emergencies/diseases/novel-coronavirus-2019/situation-reports

WHO (2020b). Naming the coronavirus disease (COVID-19) and the virus that causes it. https://www.who.int/emergencies/diseases/novel-coronavirus-2019/technical-guidance/naming-the-coronavirus-disease-(covid-2019)-and-the-virus-that-causes-it

WHO (2020c) The ACT Accelerator frequently asked questions. https://www.who.int/initiatives/act-accelerator/faq

WHO (2020d) 'Estimating Mortality from COVID-19' 4th August 2020 https://www.who.int/news-room/commentaries/detail/estimating-mortality-from-covid-19

WHO (2020e) Contact tracing in the context of COVID-19. https://www.who.int/publications/i/item/contact-tracing-in-the-context-of-covid-19]

WHO (2020f) Transmission of SARS-CoV-2:implications for infection prevention precautions. 9 July 2020 https://www.who.int/news-room/commentaries/detail/transmission-of-sars-cov-2-implications-for-infection-prevention-precautions

WIKIPEDIA (2020c) Clap for Our Carers. https://en.wikipedia.org/wiki/Clap_for_Our_Carers

Wuhan City Health Committee (WCHC 2019). Wuhan Municipal Health and Health Commission's briefing on the current pneumonia epidemic situation in our city 2019 http://wjw.wuhan.gov.cn/front/web/showDetail/2019123108989

WYATT R., (2013) Pain and ethnicity. AMA Journal of Ethics. 15 (5): 449-454https://journalofethics.ama-assn.org/article/pain-and-ethnicity/2013-05

Xiao, K., et al (2020) Isolation of SARS-C0V-2-related coronavirus from Malayan pangolins. Nature. https://doi. org/10.1038/s41586-020-2313-x (2020) https://www.nature.com/articles/s41586-020-2313-x_reference.pdf

Xing, S, Bonebrake, TC, Cheng W, Zhang, M, Ades, G, Shaw, D, Zhou, Y. Pangolins. Chapter 14. Meat and medicine: historic and contemporary use in Asia. Academic Press 2020 https://www.sciencedirect.com/science/article/pii/B9780128155073000149?via%3Dihub

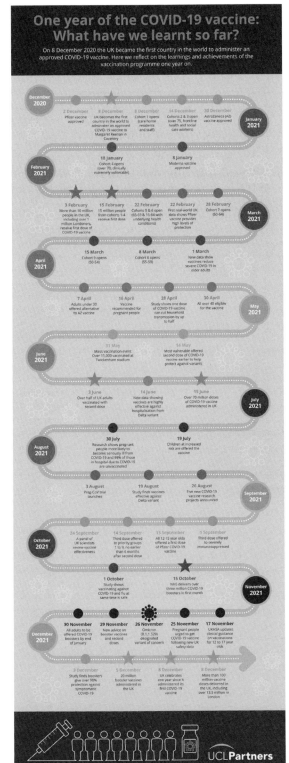

One year of the COVID-19 vaccine: what have we learnt so far? (*Vaccine timeline developed by UCLPartners and 1st impression Creative on behalf of NHS London/Public Health England's London Vaccination programme*)

About the Author

Ellen Welch is a GP based in Cumbria. She worked as remote GP during the pandemic for an NHS Out of Hours provider fielding calls from 111 – which saw a huge surge in demand particularly at the start of the crisis. She also spent much of 2020 being pregnant, and was a grateful recipient of the Covid vaccine when it was made available to healthcare workers.

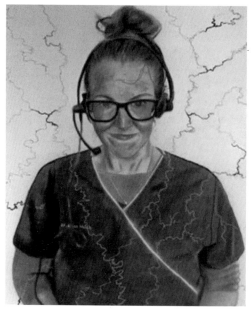

Portrait drawn during the pandemic as part of the #portraitsforNHSheroes project. (*Alex Bird. (www.facebook. com/ABirdArtist; www.instagram.com/ alexbird_drawings alexbirdartworks@ gmail.com*)